UNEXPECTED

UNEXPECTED

*A Postpartum
Survival Guide*

Erin Stevens, MD

Illustrated by Lisa Troutman

ISBN 13: 978-1-63489-319-0

Library of Congress Catalog Number: 2020902617
Printed in the United States of America
First Printing: 2020
24 23 22 21 20   5 4 3 2 1

Illustrations by Lisa Troutman
Design by Patrick Maloney

Wise Ink Creative Publishing
807 Broadway St. NE, Suite 46
Minneapolis, MN 55413
wiseink.com

To order, visit itascabooks.com or call 1-800-901-3480. Reseller discounts available.

I always told my fourth-grade teacher, Char Auge, that when I wrote a book someday, I would dedicate it to her. At the time, I was planning it to be a children's book. Life changes, but Ms. Auge's constant support and encouragement of my creativity haven't been forgotten.

This one's for you, Ms. Auge. Sorry if that's weird.

CONTENTS

Conception   8

1. I'll Be Needing Stitches   15

2. Cut. It. Out.   29

3. There Will Be Blood   43

4. Ain't Nobody Gonna Cramp My Style   51

5. If Peeing Your Pants Is Cool,
   Consider Me Miles Davis   57

6. Everybody Poops   65

7. Pain in the Butt   71

8. Working on My Fitness   77

9. Your Body Is a Wonderland   83

10. Let's Get It On   89

11. Stop in the Name of Love   95

12. Milk It for All It's Worth   107

13. Not Gonna Do It   119

14. Formula for Success   123

15. I Can't Believe I Ate the Whole Thing   131

16. Free Your Mind   143

17. I C U, BB   149

18. I Can Tell That We Are
        Going to Be Friends   155

19. I Am So Lonely   159

20. Dream a Little Dream   163

21. We're Going to Make It after All   169

22. Postpartum Survival Kit   173

23. Keep Away from the Danger   177

24. Who You Gonna Call?   181

25. Help Me If You Can   185

    Afterbirth   191

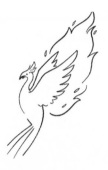

CONCEPTION

I F YOU'RE READING this, you (or someone you love) probably are or recently were pregnant. I'm going to do my best not to assume anything else about you or your experience throughout the remainder of this book. The world of health care (and the world at large) often inadvertently excludes people and obstructs needed care. I want this book to be welcoming and inclusive. As such, I will not use words such as "mother" and "mom." Not every person who experiences a pregnancy and delivery is a woman. Not every person who experiences a pregnancy and delivery considers themselves a parent (as in some cases of surrogacy, adoption, and stillbirth). Not every person who experiences a pregnancy and delivery fits into the box society has created for them. But every person who experiences a pregnancy and delivery *is* a modified version of themselves emerging from a life-changing event, just like the phoenix, the bird of Greek mythology that rises from its own ashes. Postpartum individuals are phoenixes, and that's the word I've chosen to use throughout this guide.

During pregnancy, it takes a lot of work to prepare for a baby. Depending on the circumstances, people might have multiple baby showers, work tirelessly on setting up a nursery, go on shopping sprees for adorable baby clothes, spend hours communicating with adoption agencies, coordinate each detail with the future parents for whom they're carrying the pregnancy, plan for neonatal surgery or special pediatric care for known problems with the baby, or make decisions regarding interventions versus neonatal hospice for truly grave diagnoses.

But what about you? How prepared are you for what happens to YOU after delivery?

As an OB/GYN physician, I've noticed that somewhere in all the preparation for the time after delivery, the phoenix gets lost. Expectations for postpartum recovery are veiled in secrecy by the stifling power of cute little bows and animal-themed burp cloths. Childbirth and the postpartum state are romanticized, and there's a strong societal expectation that the time after delivery is strictly glorious and wonderful. Most phoenixes – even those with the most straightforward, medically uncomplicated circumstances – have no idea what to expect for themselves, how to manage normal postpartum issues, or what is abnormal or concerning. Not only is this unacceptable, but it's dangerous too.

When I graduated from residency training and entered private practice, I began seeing patients more consistently in postpartum follow-up. I realized our medical community is failing phoenixes. On a broader scale, we know that the United States is the only developed nation with a rising maternal mortality rate and that the incidence of many medical complications is increasing in pregnancy and the postpartum period. There are myriad contributors to this, not all of which have been fully identified and explored. Risks aren't equal for all populations and can be impacted by unjust elements such as differences in health insurance, decreasing obstetric services in rural areas, and implicit bias. Typical pregnancy and postpartum care is designed for cisgender, heterosexual, white, healthy women with viable, planned pregnancies who live in resource-rich settings. Phoenixes of color, for instance, are more likely to die than their white counterparts, which is certainly influenced by systemic racial discrimination and stereotyping. Even simple Google image searches for "pregnancy" or "postpartum" produce results overwhelmingly featuring white women cradling their term pregnant bellies or healthy babies.

It's common for patients to report that their mental and physical health concerns are overlooked or ignored. In 2017, tennis superstar Serena Williams recognized and reported the symptoms of a pulmonary embolism (a blood clot in her lungs) during her postpartum recovery and still had to fight her way to the appropriate workup and management. The singer Adele is one of many celebrities who have publicly shared their experiences with postpartum depression to raise awareness, yet mental health stigma can hold phoenixes back from acknowledging and addressing symptoms. Phoenixes of all races, backgrounds, socioeconomic statuses, locations, and pregnancy experiences need to know what is and isn't normal in order to confidently discuss their concerns and advocate for themselves in the medical field. We in the health care system certainly have to get our act together, but I want you to know: *you are allowed to care about your health, and you deserve compassionate attention and answers.*

Recognizing the postpartum problem both directly in front of me and nationwide, I wanted to do my part to make things better. Unfortunately, my training hadn't done much to prepare me to help. The world of obstetrics is focused on getting you through the pregnancy and delivery. After that, a majority of our experience with the postpartum period is related to severe complications that lead to prolonged or repeated hospitalization. There's a perception that the "normal stuff" is easy and everyone can just figure it out.

So, I sought assistance from — where else? — social media. I posted on Facebook, Twitter, and Reddit in search of advice. Thank you to my friends and family, my colleagues, and the anonymous strangers of the internet for their contributions to this guide. This wouldn't be possible without you. I learned so much, and I hope together we can help every phoenix achieve postpartum success.

The following pages include summaries of expectations and recommendations for specific subject areas, sprinkled with quotations and anecdotes from real phoenixes. Most sections end with some combination of Warnings, Questions, and Supplies. The Warnings are reasons to seek medical care, the Questions are thoughts to help guide conversation with a health care clinician, and the Supplies are items to buy (or put on a registry) in preparation for recovery.

Do not use this guide as your sole source of medical advice. I want to help everyone as best I can, but there's no way I could include information about what to do in every possible circumstance for every possible phoenix in every possible place, especially while trying to keep this book relatively short and sweet (as sweet as real talk about the postpartum experience can be). Your experience with a topic in this book may fall outside the realm of what I discuss, or maybe a topic you're concerned about isn't mentioned here. That doesn't invalidate your experience with that issue or mean it's not important. This guide is meant to be a supplement to the care you receive from your own doctor, midwife, nurse practitioner, physician assistant, or other health care professional.

Whatever happens, never lose sight of the fact that growing a human inside of you and then going through the process of getting it outside of you is a difficult, dangerous, and tremendous feat. Know and own your strength and greatness.

> *Ice packs are your best friend for WEEKS!*

Kristen, Pennsylvania

1

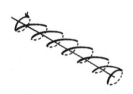

I'LL BE NEEDING STITCHES

Tearing with Vaginal Delivery

THE SECOND QUESTION I typically hear on the receiving end of a vaginal delivery is "How much did I tear?" (The first is "How much does the baby weigh?", as if I somehow cleverly inserted a scale into the abdomen or chest of the phoenix, where I usually set the baby.) Often, I pause before replying because if the answer isn't "Not at all" or "Not much," it can be difficult to word the response palatably. Phoenixes are very interested in the vaginal aftermath of their efforts.

Tearing is common with vaginal deliveries and often requires stitches, but the thought of this can promote a lot of predelivery anxiety. The fear of tearing and other potential consequences is what I see as the main driver of requests for elective Cesarean delivery. It would be silly to tell you not to think about it, but I hate seeing patients stressing out and letting it frame their entire mindset heading into delivery. Tearing is generally not the end of the world.

As with many issues in the medical world, prevention is key. Tearing risk can be reduced with a few measures. Try perineal massage starting at thirty-five to thirty-six weeks of pregnancy. To do this, you — or, more likely, an intimate buddy — will use a lubricant (an over-the-counter lubricant marketed for use with sex is fine, or you can use vitamin E, coconut, or olive oil) to massage and stretch the tissue at the bottom of the opening of your vagina a couple times per day. Massage for fifteen seconds, then take a break for a similar duration. Repeat this pattern for a few minutes each time. This will cause some discomfort due to the sensitivity of the tissues, but it shouldn't cause pain. My colleagues and I have seen patients in early pregnancy who have already started perineal massage. This is not necessary, probably uncomfortable, and a drain on your time. If you're cool with that and it makes you feel better to do it, by all means, carry on. Otherwise, focus on other hobbies until you're closer to delivery.

If it is deemed medically safe to do so, you may

be able to spend at least the early part of labor in a bathtub at home or at your delivery facility, if available. Laboring in water might reduce severe tearing, although the studies on this could be muddied by other factors. Some centers are equipped for water births (actually delivering and not just laboring in a tub). This is not recommended by the American College of Obstetricians and Gynecologists (ACOG), which provides guidelines for all aspects of OB/GYN care in the United States and beyond. ACOG's official recommendation is that "birth occur on land, not in water." (It doesn't mention a thing about delivering in the air, but I don't think the world is ready for drone delivery yet.) Water birth is popular at many birth centers and some hospitals. If you are hoping to labor or deliver in water, talk to your prenatal care/delivery clinician to see if this would be safe or possible for you in your particular circumstances. Please make sure you are in clean water if you do this — don't go jump in a lake.

Try perineal massage starting at thirty-five to thirty-six weeks of pregnancy.

Copious mineral oil or other lubricant can be applied to the vulvar and vaginal tissues while you push and while the baby emerges. The hospitals where I work supply delivery rooms with tiny packets of lubricant, and I always ask the nurse working with me for all of them. Fans of the TV show *Parks and Recreation* might recall a scene where Ron Swanson orders "all the bacon and eggs" at a restaurant. "I'm worried what you just heard was, 'Give me a lot of bacon and eggs.' What I said was, 'Give me all the bacon and eggs you have,'" he says. This is how I feel about lube packets. You can bring your own mineral oil to your delivery just in case tiny lube packets are the only thing available at the facility where you deliver.

Avoiding unnecessary interventions and optimizing your and your clinician's control during delivery can also help to avoid tearing. As the baby's head comes down lower, your pain and pressure become increasingly intense. The stretching of your tissue peaks, a point some people call the "ring of fire" because it burns, burns, burns. As difficult as it is, this is a key point to keep your head in the game — walk the line, if you will — and focus on steady pushing. Your delivery clinician can gently guide the baby's head in the appropriate direction for a smooth arrival that causes less trauma to your tissues.

Sometimes, though, tearing is unavoidable. If you think about the path the baby takes to bust into the world, you can imagine there are many areas for potential tearing. One of the most common sites is the area between the bottom of the vaginal opening and the anus called the perineum, which can give way as the baby emerges. Perineal tearing is categorized from the first through fourth degree, depending on how deep it goes (skin, muscle, anal sphincter, rectal tissue). A fourth-degree perineal laceration is your worst-case scenario with potentially long-lasting effects, and it is a major fear of many phoenixes when thinking about a vaginal delivery.

Sometimes, tearing is unavoidable.

Other categories of tearing include labial (lips), vaginal (inner genital tissue), periurethral (around the hole you pee from), periclitoral (around the sensitive bundle of nerve fibers that often provides pleasure with sexual activity), and cervical (the opening to the uterus/womb). Whoever helps deliver the baby should thoroughly evaluate all these areas to see if tearing has occurred.

I do my best to carefully control all factors and provide protection during delivery, but sometimes the baby will suddenly begin emerging faster than anticipated, maybe even with a fist next to its face, punching its way out, wreaking havoc along the way. This is a common theme in obstetrics — no matter how much we prepare, the baby might have its own plan.

Risk of tearing can increase for phoenixes who

ANATOMY for POTENTIAL STITCH PLACEMENT

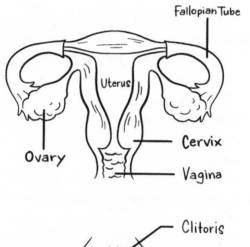

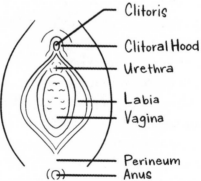

have never experienced a delivery before, those with very large babies, babies in unusual delivery positions (such as "sunny-side up," otherwise known as occiput posterior position), or those whose deliveries require assistance from devices such as forceps and vacuum extractors.

> **SIDE NOTE:** I know the word "vacuum" creates an awful mental picture in this setting, but we are not talking about a Hoover. It's a gentle suction cup–like apparatus that should probably be referred to by its other name (ventouse) or some other term to decrease how scary it sounds. Forceps doesn't sound great either. I was taught to describe forceps as large, gentle spoons, as if using giant silverware on a baby is more comforting. Forceps or a vacuum extractor may be recommended to expedite delivery in certain circumstances, including concern for the baby's well-being.

Historically, episiotomies — making a small cut at the vaginal opening with a surgical instrument — used to be quite common. They were thought to help deliveries move along more easily and reduce overall tearing. Studies haven't supported those assumptions, however. Episiotomies often don't heal as well as natural tearing, and sometimes they can create a path for *worsened* tearing, especially in the perineal region. When progress in a delivery is slow, rarely is that particular tissue the problem. The general practice now is to avoid episiotomy. Your delivery clinician might recommend or emergently perform an episiotomy based on specific circumstances. If this happens, make sure that person debriefs with you.

> The general practice now is to avoid episiotomy.

If tearing occurs, stitches may or may not be needed. Stitches help stop bleeding and bring tissue back to its normal anatomical position so everything heals correctly. Sometimes tears are relatively superficial (such as skinning your knee by falling off a bike), though, and don't bleed significantly. Placing stitches around tears like that may be more problematic than just leaving them alone.

You only want stitches where truly necessary. You may have heard stories about the husband stitch, one or two extra stitches placed at the vagina's opening in a grossly patriarchal attempt to narrow it due to a perception by certain clinicians of future sexual benefit to a partner with a penis. Most times, phoenixes aren't even aware this is being done to them. Ensure your clinician communicates with you so you don't end up with stitches where they're not needed.

Stitches are often placed in the delivery room. Sometimes phoenixes need to be brought to the operating room so they can be made more comfortable and so all areas can be appropriately visualized to ensure the safest repair of the tears. Believe me, you want to make sure whoever is placing the stitches can evaluate everything completely for correct and complete repair.

Often, numbing medication is injected before stitching. If you have an epidural, you might not need this. If you don't have an epidural, you definitely will need it. The injection of numbing medication typically causes a short burning sensation, but you shouldn't feel much pain after that. Without any pain control, it is incredibly difficult for a phoenix to stay relaxed and motionless enough to safely repair all tearing in order to stop the bleeding and ensure appropriate healing.

Almost always, the type of suture used will absorb on its own over several weeks, and you will not have to have it removed. If your delivery clinician doesn't specify this, make sure you ask. Just because the stitches don't require removal doesn't mean you don't have to return for evaluation after delivery, however. When a patient experiences significant tearing, I have them return to the office earlier than I would otherwise recommend for a routine postpartum appointment so I can examine the area and make sure it is healing properly.

Many phoenixes ask, "How many stitches did I get?" This can be difficult to answer. In some cases, the suture at the site of each tear is placed in a manner similar to sewing, continuing in what we call a running fashion, rather than being placed in a series of individual knots. Instead of focusing on how many, I discuss with the patient where their tearing was anatomically located and which tears needed stitches. Make sure someone has a similar conversation with you.

The site(s) of tearing will feel tender throughout the course of healing. Swelling will also likely accompany the tearing. Your bits will be uncomfortable even when you are sedentary, and friction will likely cause you more discomfort when walking and performing other normal everyday activities.

Ibuprofen and acetaminophen can help with

TYPES of STITCHES
(almost always absorbable)

Continuous
Sutures (Running)

Interrupted or
Intermittent

discomfort but might not take away the pain completely (please follow dosing instructions and make sure you don't have any contraindications to these medications). Witch hazel and perineal spray will be your friends.

> **PRO TIP:** Spritz one of these products on overnight pads and keep them in the freezer to use when needed for extra soothing effect. Ice packs and Tucks pads (medicated pads generally used for hemorrhoids) are marketed for this purpose as well, but some phoenixes do not like the texture of these. Sitting in a warm, shallow bath — with Epsom salt, if you'd like (this is called a sitz bath) — can be comforting. You may need to sit on a pillow or cushion, or avoid sitting for long periods for weeks. Using a spray bottle after urination (your own handheld bidet!) and patting to dry can decrease the burning of urine contacting the sites of tearing and decrease the trauma of wiping to the sensitive healing tissue.

Luckily, these areas tend to heal well in the long run. Sometimes a daily personal lubricant or estrogen cream may be needed to help with the discomfort and healing of the process. This can be especially helpful in the setting of lactation because estrogen stimulation of the vaginal tissues is decreased during that time. Estrogen creams can unfortunately be expensive and are not often covered by insurance. Talk to your obstetric clinician about recommendations for this.

If you notice a bad vaginal odor, greenish discharge,

or severe pain that is intolerable despite oral medications, something is likely wrong. A phoenix once told
me she was unable to walk and had green discharge
postpartum. She was exhausted from lack of sleep,
focused on her baby, and unaware
of signs of infection, so she as-
sumed this was part of the normal
healing process. She dealt with
the symptoms and unnecessarily
suffered for weeks before being
evaluated at her doctor's office and diagnosed with
an infection. Her symptoms improved considerably
once she was appropriately treated. Besides the frus-
tration of the acute symptoms of infection, untreated
infection can lead to inadequate or abnormal healing,
so it's in your best interest to address any suspicion
of it with a medical professional as soon as possible.

Luckily, these areas tend to heal well in the long run.

In rare circumstances, the tissue simply doesn't
heal appropriately, which can cause horrible long-
term complications such as persistent pain, loss
of control of urine or bowel movements, urine or
bowel coming out through the vagina, or consistent
abnormal discharge or bleeding. Improper healing is
more likely if there is undiagnosed infection, if the
phoenix has a medical issue that interferes with normal healing, or if the original tearing wasn't repaired

correctly. Some phoenixes ultimately need surgery to remedy this situation.

Bottom line: don't ignore anything you see or feel down below that doesn't seem right.

WARNINGS
- Bad vaginal odor
- Greenish discharge
- Loss of control of urine or bowel movements
- Severe pain

QUESTIONS
- Is everything healing correctly?
- What kind of stitches were used?
- What kind of tearing do I have?
- What should I do to promote healing?
- What symptoms might I notice from the tearing?

SUPPLIES
- Acetaminophen
- Epsom salt
- Ibuprofen
- Ice packs
- Pillow
- Spray bottle
- Tucks pads
- Witch hazel

"Natural childbirth" denotes vaginal delivery, leaving some moms who deliver via C-section feeling like they didn't do it naturally. All childbirth is natural, and if we're talking about how the baby actually came out of mom's body, it's either a vaginal delivery or a C-section. I understand shorthand references are easier, but they really do set up a dichotomy where a mom who births naturally is doing it right and a mom who does it differently isn't.

Julia, Minnesota

2

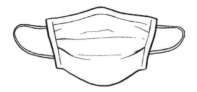

CUT. IT. OUT.

Cesarean Section Implications

OME BABIES ENTER the world vaginally. Some don't. If you look around any given room of people, can you tell who was delivered vaginally and who was delivered by Cesarean section? Sure can't.

Delivery by Cesarean section (C-section) doesn't make the delivery or the love and sacrifice of the whole process any different in quality. A C-section is not "less than" a vaginal delivery. It doesn't make a delivery unnatural. (Overall, I would love if people stopped using the term "natural" when discussing pregnancy, labor, delivery, and the postpartum period.) C-section is simply a mode of delivery that is one of the potential outcomes of a pregnancy.

Cesarean section is one of the most common surgical procedures in the world, so most OB/GYNs are very skilled at it. In the time it takes you to watch an episode of your favorite TV sitcom, most of us could complete a C-section and sit down with you and some popcorn to see the ending. If we scheduled every pregnant person for a C-section right off the bat instead of having them go through the process of labor and potential vaginal delivery, it would be more efficient for everyone involved. So why do we generally recommend attempting vaginal delivery in cases where it is safe to do so?

Although C-sections are common, they are still major surgeries that come with risks to consider and weigh against those of vaginal delivery (no delivery is risk free). C-section risks exist for the phoenix, the baby, and future pregnancies.

C-SECTION RISKS

- The phoenix will likely have increased bleeding with a C-section, compared to a vaginal delivery.

- Sometimes bleeding from any kind of delivery is significant enough to require additional medications or procedures. This sometimes includes hysterectomy (complete removal of the uterus), an outcome that is more common — but remains rare — after C-section than vaginal delivery. Even if you are considering hysterectomy anyway, this is more dangerous if it occurs immediately after delivery due to the greatly increased blood flow to the uterus at this time.

- Any surgery comes with the risk of infection. Antibiotics are administered for any C-section, but they cannot completely eliminate that risk. Infection can develop inside the uterus, surrounding the uterus, or in the layers of the abdominal wall. Mild infections of the skin can be treated with antibiotics by mouth. Severe infections in deeper tissues may require IV antibiotics, another surgery, or the placement of drains.

- We have to be gentle not to harm areas such as the bowel or the bladder next to the uterus. Phoenixes who have had previous surgeries, including previous C-sections, might have significant scar tissue, which increases the procedure's difficulty and risk for potential injury to these areas. Injury to the bladder usually can be repaired with stitches, and the phoenix often needs to leave the hospital with a catheter (a tube that drains urine) in place for a short time. Injury to the bowel cannot always be simply repaired, and sometimes a portion of the bowel needs to be removed.

- We have to be careful that none of the surgical instruments or required delivery maneuvers hurt the baby. In even the most controlled, cautious C-sections, a baby might be cut with an instrument.

- With each C-section, there is a further increased risk in future pregnancies of uterine rupture, where the wall of the uterus comes open during labor, which is life-threatening to a phoenix and a baby.

- With each C-section, there is a further increased risk in future pregnancies of placental growth in abnormal locations. The placenta can actually grow into and through the scar from a previous C-section. It can grow into the bladder and/or bowel, requiring not only a hysterectomy at the time of delivery but sometimes removal of a portion of the bladder or bowel. That's not an optimal circumstance for anyone.

Of course, going through a C-section avoids the vaginal tearing and potential related complications reviewed in the previous chapter. It avoids the potential of a baby becoming stuck during a vaginal delivery (called "shoulder dystocia"), which is more common with very large babies, babies with large abdomens compared to their heads, phoenixes who have gestational diabetes, or phoenixes who have had a shoulder dystocia before. A C-section may be recommended based on the baby's position, the placenta's location, previous surgical history, the delivery's urgency, or the labor's progress, among other indications.

In all deliveries, no matter how they are accomplished, the top priority is health and safety. Ultimately, you have agency over what happens to your body. Some phoenixes may elect for a C-section after discussing risks and benefits compared to vaginal delivery. Some phoenixes go through pregnancy dead set on delivering vaginally and can be distressed when discussing C-section. Often, patients who have prioritized vaginal delivery start crying once I introduce the conversation about potential C-section. It can be heartbreaking to see. Thorough counseling about the clinical situation can help reduce some of these negative emotions. If a C-section is recommended, make sure you un-

> In all deliveries, no matter how they are accomplished, the top priority is health and safety.

derstand why and what the implications would be if a C-section weren't performed.

A phoenix who had an unplanned C-section once told me about how she felt like her body had failed her and that she had done something wrong. It took her months to come to terms with the experience. Grappling with the circumstances made her post-partum experience more difficult, and she wished her OB had prepared and educated her more regarding the possibility for C-section, as well as the implications for recovery.

No matter the reason C-section is pursued, its recovery is different than a vaginal delivery. It will likely require you to spend more time in the hospital and have more pain. Talk to your delivery clinician and the anesthesiologist involved in the C-section about what measures may be taken to reduce your postpartum pain. Take the pain medications you need! I have seen a lot of patients struggle with pain in the early days of recovery because they wanted to avoid taking opioid medications. While I can understand the fear of side effects and dependency, uncontrolled pain can complicate recovery. Take your prescribed non-narcotic pain medications scheduled around the clock initially, then take whatever harder-hitting medications are available to you for pain that's still not controlled after that.

Your mobility and activities will be more restricted after a C-section than after a vaginal delivery, as the large incision requires a lot of caution to heal appropriately. Trust me, you do not want to overdo it. An incision that comes open — in any of the layers, not just the skin layer that you can see — can be a big problem. Wearing an abdominal binder can help decrease discomfort and increase support while the layers heal.

LAYERS of a C-SECTION

Skin
Subcutaneous Fat
Fascia
Muscle
Peritoneum
Uterine Wall
Amniotic Sac

- **Skin:** This is the only incision you're going to see. Usually, it's in a bikini line horizontal location, and less often it is right down the middle of your lower belly. Usually, this is closed with stitches, but sometimes staples are used instead.

- **Subcutaneous fat:** Everyone has some fat beneath the skin; don't worry about it. Sometimes stitches are placed in this layer to prevent fluid buildup (called a seroma) that can become infected.

- **Fascia:** A fibrous tissue that surrounds your abdominal muscles. This is put back together with stitches.

- **Muscle:** This is not usually cut, but sometimes it needs to be in order to obtain better access to the uterus. In this case, it is loosely reapproximated with stitches (stitching it together too tightly will not be good in the long run). Recovery might be more difficult and painful if incisions are made into the muscles.

- **Peritoneum:** A membrane that covers your organs. This may or may not be stitched closed.

- **Uterine wall:** The uterus has a few layers, but the main idea is that the womb needs to be entered to get to the baby. Similar to the skin incision, this incision is typically horizontal in the lower part of the uterus, but sometimes it needs to be created vertically either in the upper or lower part of the uterus. The type of incision may determine if you can try for a vaginal delivery in the future if you wish. This incision will be stitched closed, and the area where it was made will be weaker than the rest of the uterus's muscle wall.

- **Amniotic sac:** The membranous layer containing the fluid around the baby (all this tissue should come out with delivery).

During the first six weeks after a C-section, do not jump back into your exercise routine. Avoid creating increased pressure within your abdomen, as that places tension on the stitches. Walking and gentle movements are okay. During this time, also try to avoid going up and down stairs, and lifting more than ten to fifteen pounds.

You should not drive for the first week after a C-section, or during any time that you are taking narcotic medications. Before you set out on the road, practice quickly slamming on the brakes in your garage, driveway, or parking lot. Your leg's ability to respond and move appropriately might be impaired from the surgery's impact on nerves and muscles, which could be dangerous out among other cars.

Keep the incision clean by letting warm, soapy water run over it in the shower and patting it to dry. Don't scrub hard or rub the incision to dry until your health care clinician has confirmed that the skin has closed. Do not soak the incision in water – that means no baths with water to the level of the incision, no swimming, and no hot tubs.

If the top of your pants irritates the incision, tuck a large menstrual pad between the incision and your pants for cushioning. Try not to touch the incision too much, and make sure your hands are completely clean if you do. Many phoenixes become fixated on using lotions or creams on it. Clear any topical agents with your obstetrics clinician, and realize that you may be introducing bacteria into your incision each time you apply.

Aside from the pain from surgery, you are likely to notice other sensations along and around the incision. You might experience burning, tingling, or numbness due to nerve irritation. This often resolves over time, but that can take weeks, months, or even years for some phoenixes.

The mindset "Once a C-section, always a C-section" is largely a thing of the past. Depending on the circumstances surrounding pregnancy and delivery, some phoenixes who have previously had one to two C-sections are safely able to deliver vaginally with future pregnancies if they choose. Discuss your particular circumstances with your prenatal care clinician. If you have had a C-section in one pregnancy and prefer to have a C-section again with the next, this is generally scheduled in the thirty-ninth week of pregnancy — but it may be earlier, depending on the circumstances of your previous C-section as well as your current pregnancy.

WARNINGS

- Discharge or bleeding from the incision

- Inability to have a bowel movement

- Pain not controlled with prescribed medications

- Persistent vomiting

- Separation of the skin incision

QUESTIONS

- Can I try for a vaginal delivery in the future if I want to?

- How should I care for my incision?

- Is my incision healing correctly?

- Was there anything unusual or noteworthy found or done during my C-section that I should know (such as encountering lots of scar tissue, having to cut extra tissue, performing additional procedures)?

- What activity restrictions do I have?

- What kind of C-section incision do I have on the uterus?

SUPPLIES

- Abdominal binder

- Acetaminophen

- Heating pad

- Ibuprofen

- Menstrual pad (to decrease friction on the incision)

- Prescribed pain medications

I had my husband run to get large overnight pads for after I ran out of the ones the hospital gave me. I wish I had known so I was more stocked at home. I just didn't realize how much you bleed afterwards!

Abby, Minnesota

3

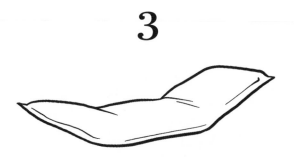

THERE WILL BE BLOOD

Bleeding

A HUMAN JUST came out of your body. Oh, yes, there will be blood.

The mixture of blood, discharge, and tissue that comes out of your uterus after delivery is called lochia (from a Greek word meaning "of childbirth"). To return to normal, your uterus needs to get all that stuff out of it. Think of this as a horrible, extended cleanse.

The amount and duration of lochia can vary for each phoenix. Generally, it starts at its reddest and heaviest over the first few days. When I say heaviest, think of your bloodiest period, then add some extra blood with a side of blood. The bleeding will taper over time. Typically, it will be followed by brownish or pinkish discharge, then whitish or yellowish discharge. Your bleeding and discharge may wax and wane, often for up to the first six weeks.

> Think of your bloodiest period, and then add some extra blood with a side of blood.

One phoenix told me she had no idea what to expect with lochia. She was told to stock up on pads, so she knew there would be some bleeding. She was caught off guard when she experienced what seemed like months' worth of periods pouring out as blood and clots. This led to an embarrassing situation when she was shopping at Target while not fully prepared with the appropriate menstrual products. She stopped her intended shopping, quickly purchased a pair of sweatpants and a package of pads, took care of the situation in the store bathroom, then completed her planned shopping.

You should not use tampons or menstrual cups during the first six weeks after delivery to avoid infection and improper healing. Stock up on pads of all sizes, as well as pantyliners. You're initially going to want overnight pads at all times. Change your pads or liners every couple hours, even if they are not saturated.

You'll want to wear "granny panties" that you'll feel okay throwing away. Now is not the time for any of Victoria's secrets — the less stylish your undies, the better. You want to be as comfortable as possible without worrying about the damage of any leaks. Some phoenixes choose to wear adult diapers — depends (see what I did there?) on what feels right to you. Most hospitals will provide at least one pair of mesh panties to you, which, as odd as it sounds, a lot of phoenixes love. You can purchase more pairs online at a relatively low price and enjoy them as long as you'd like.

> Some phoenixes choose to wear adult diapers.

You are bleeding too much if you persistently soak through a pad in less than an hour or two, or if you are passing clots larger than the size of lemons (if life gives you lemons, please call your obstetrics clinician). Note that if you sit for a long period of time and then stand up, you are likely to see some clots due to collected blood — this is different than the spontaneous passage of clots. Don't panic. If you're somewhat up and about, though, and all of a sudden you notice citrus-sized gobs, give your obstetrics clinician a call.

Daily bleeding and spotting that continues after the first six weeks is unusual. This might be a sign of a problem, such as retained tissue from the delivery within the uterus, and it should be evaluated. One phoenix continued bleeding daily like a light period for more than six weeks after her delivery, but she was afraid to ask if this was normal. Due to family commitments, she had to delay her routine six-week postpartum appointment at her physician's office, so she didn't have a chance to address this for a while. When she finally came in for assessment, an ultrasound showed some retained pregnancy tissue at the top of her uterus. A quick procedure removed the tissue, and she no longer experienced bleeding.

If your discharge is green or has a bad odor, these are signs of infection. If left untreated, infections in the uterus can spread to your bloodstream and make you very ill, necessitate surgery, and/or compromise your future ability to conceive.

It's atypical for bleeding to completely resolve and then return heavily. Generally, there's more of a transition. The exception to this is if your period returns. This is likely to happen earlier — even within the first six weeks — for those who are not exclusively breast- or chestfeeding, but it can happen to anyone. Talk to your obstetrics clinician if you're unsure.

On that note, your first few periods may be

irregular in timing, especially if you are breast- or chestfeeding. If your periods haven't normalized after a few months without lactating, get that checked out.

Your periods may be forever changed after delivery. It is not uncommon for people to have heavier, crampier periods long-term after childbirth. You may have to adjust to a new normal, and methods you once successfully used for controlling menstrual symptoms might not work as well anymore. Address any changes in your bleeding patterns with your gynecologist regardless, however, to determine if additional assessment is required.

WARNINGS

- Bleeding regularly beyond six weeks postpartum

- Consistently bleeding through more than one pad in an hour

- Greenish, bad-smelling discharge

- Passing clots larger than the size of lemons

- Sudden onset of heavy bleeding after bleeding has previously subsided

QUESTIONS

- Is my bleeding level normal?

- My periods are different now —
  should I be worried?

- When should I call the office about bleeding?

SUPPLIES

- Adult diapers

- Overnight menstrual pads

- Pantyliners

- Regular menstrual pads

- Throwaway underwear

> *The pains after delivery*
> *when breastfeeding*
> *can be as bad as labor.*

Maeta, Minnesota

4

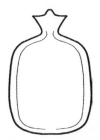

AIN'T NOBODY
GONNA CRAMP MY STYLE

Cramping

AS A CRUEL joke of nature, your uterus is going to continue contracting after delivery. It was large enough to hold the baby, feeling like it was up to your throat. It needs to get back down to its normal size and shape, usually over about six weeks, and it wants you to be aware of its presence every step of the way. Some phoenixes say the after-delivery contractions are worse than labor or the pain of delivery itself — just what you wanted to hear! At least during labor and delivery there's a clearer endpoint. Sometimes the after-delivery cramping can feel endless.

After the big contraction pains stop (within about two to three days of delivery), your uterus will continue cramping. This can range from a dull, irritating cramp to the worst period cramps of your life.

> Some phoenixes say the after-delivery contractions are worse than labor.

Cramping generally increases with nipple stimulation (whether for milk production or for fun) due to the release of the hormone oxytocin (the love hormone), which stimulates uterine contractility. While it can be helpful to mentally prepare and potentially time pain control measures around nipple stimulation, you can't prevent this from happening.

One phoenix told me she had such intense postpartum cramping that her sister-in-law started calling 911. The phoenix hung up the phone and instead squeezed her sister's hand as she yelled through it. Her sister-in-law was a little perplexed and probably scared off from having a baby anytime soon.

Ibuprofen helps best with cramping pain, though unfortunately it may not even touch the initial postdelivery contractions. You can alternate ibuprofen and acetaminophen (please follow dosing instructions on the packaging and make sure you don't have any contraindications to these medications) to gain better pain control. Opioid medications don't typically help with this kind of pain, so please be cautious with any such measures.

Heating pads applied to the belly or lower back can be helpful. If you don't have a heating pad, fill an old sock with rice and microwave it for about a minute. Make sure it feels soothing but not too hot. Whatever you use for heating, periodically check the skin beneath it to ensure you're not burning yourself.

Avoid constipation or letting your bladder stay full for long periods. Go to the bathroom regularly, including prior to going to sleep. Reducing the pressure in your nearby organs can reduce the intensity of your uterine cramping.

Have your partner or a buddy massage your abdomen and lower back. Let's be honest, this is probably a great plan regardless of whether you are having cramps. Of course, you can go to the pros for this too, but nothing beats free in-home services.

Sometimes all you can do to mildly improve cramping is curl up in the fetal position and wait it out. I suppose that's fitting, given the circumstances. Just go with it. Do what you need to do.

> Sometimes all you can do to mildly improve cramping is curl up in the fetal position.

If your pain is severe, persistent, and not alleviated by any of these measures, discuss it with your obstetrics clinician. You may have an infection or have retained blood or tissue that would need to be medically or surgically addressed.

WARNINGS

- Pain not controlled with oral medications

- Sudden onset of severe pain after pain previously improved

QUESTIONS

- Is my pain level normal?

- What can I take or do to help?

SUPPLIES

- Acetaminophen

- Heating pad

- Ibuprofen

Incontinence is an unfortunately common thing. It will get better. It's helpful just being aware. Have Poise pads and Depends.

Casey, Delaware

5

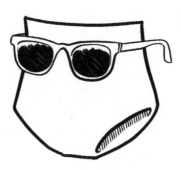

IF PEEING YOUR PANTS IS COOL, CONSIDER ME MILES DAVIS

Incontinence and Other Urinary Issues

SOMEONE BOUNCED AROUND in your pelvis for months and then forcibly emerged from your body. Your muscles, bladder, and urethra might not be happy about that. Many phoenixes require catheterization (placing a tube through your urethra into your bladder to drain urine when you're unable to pee on your own, or when it's important not to have a physically full bladder) at some point in their delivery and postpartum course, and that can impact initial urinary function too.

Urination will feel uncomfortable right away. Pee regularly to prevent your bladder from becoming too stretched and tense and to prevent increasing discomfort in your pelvis. If you have persistent pain with urination, particularly burning at the urethra (the external hole where the urine comes out), you may need to be evaluated for a urinary tract infection (UTI). Note that if you experienced any vaginal tearing with delivery, the sites of tearing are likely to burn during urination simply due to urine irritating the extra-sensitive healing tissue.

You might start feeling like a baby yourself in that you have seemingly no control over when you're peeing. You might notice urine leakage when you cough, laugh, or sneeze – this is called stress incontinence. You might notice urine leakage when you have a strong sensation that you need to pee and don't make it to the bathroom in time – this is urge incontinence. Or you might notice urine leakage at any old time. Even after your postpartum bleeding stops, you will likely want to continue wearing a pad or liner to protect from leaks. Incontinence pads and liners are made for this purpose and hold urine more adequately than menstrual pads and liners. This is important to avoid oversaturating the pads, which can irritate your skin.

> You might start feeling like a baby yourself in that you have seemingly no control over when you're peeing.

Urine leakage can be embarrassing, which prevents most phoenixes from talking about it. Often, it takes a lot of prying for patients to admit to me that they are "having some dribbling." Please know this issue is common and you are not alone, even if you've never heard a friend or family member talk about it.

One phoenix did not realize loss of urine could be a postpartum issue. Thinking she was having some sort of abnormal vaginal discharge, she wore menstrual pantyliners, which in turn contributed to vulvar irritation and itching. This convinced her the problem was a persistent yeast infection, and she used over-the-counter Monistat multiple times before undergoing evaluation for an appropriate diagnosis. She switched to incontinence liners, started timing bathroom breaks more frequently, and stopped using Monistat unnecessarily. With time, her incontinence wasn't an issue anymore.

For the most part, leakage will improve over time, but it may never completely resolve. Risks for long-term incontinence are similar between phoenixes who deliver vaginally and phoenixes who deliver via C-section.

Kegel exercises (contracting the muscles of your pelvic floor — the ones that surround your vagina) can be helpful to decrease leaking. Squeeze the muscles you would use to stop urination mid-stream or to pick something up with your vagina (as we are all prone to doing). It's kind of hard to do, right? Many people do Kegel exercises incorrectly. It takes work.

Many people do Kegel exercises incorrectly.

Pelvic floor physical therapy is an excellent resource. This is a subset of physical therapy that focuses on the muscles surrounding the vagina. A pelvic floor physical therapist can help you do Kegel exercises correctly and strengthen your pelvic muscles overall. Sometimes they will use a biofeedback device to show you the activity of your muscles throughout the exercises. Many patients are initially hesitant to try pelvic floor physical therapy due to feeling awkward about it but are happy they did it once they get over the hurdle of trepidation. A lot of my patients have noticed significant improvement in urine leakage with this intervention.

A couple medications help with urge incontinence. These medications can impact milk production and can have side effects for the phoenix that must be considered. Talk to your gynecologist if you think you need them.

Silicone devices called pessaries support the urethra and can help in some cases of incontinence. They can be cumbersome but are an option if your symptoms are persistent and intolerable. There are also over-the-counter disposable urethral supports that are placed almost like a tampon. Not everyone loves the way these feel, but it is another option if you are frustrated with your symptoms.

Some phoenixes for whom incontinence is a persistent problem may be candidates for surgical management. Surgery is deferred until completion of childbearing, so if you're thinking about pregnancy again in the future, this isn't the best option yet.

You may also have the opposite problem of incontinence — instead of peeing when you don't necessarily want to, not being able to pee when you do. This is not great either, and it could be related to neurological issues, infection, trauma or injury to the bladder or urethra, or compression of the bladder from a distended uterus or portion of the bowels. This problem is hard to ignore because it will cause you significant pain to have a completely filled bladder that can't be emptied. See a health care clinician right away.

WARNINGS

- Blood in urine

- Constant urine leakage

- Inability to urinate

- Persistent burning pain with urination

QUESTIONS

- Do you have recommendations for a pelvic floor physical therapist?

- Is the change I'm noticing to my urinary habits normal?

- Is there anything I can or should do for incontinence at this point?

SUPPLIES

- Incontinence pantyliners

A common side effect of any pain medicine is constipation, and after getting stitches, that first week I was terrified to go. I was in so much pain!

Mattie, Minnesota

6

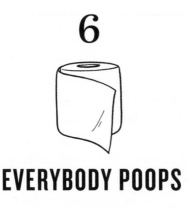

EVERYBODY POOPS

Constipation

IT'S TERRIFYING AND traumatic, but it has to happen sometime: the first poop after delivery. Many phoenixes tell me this is the most painful part of postpartum recovery.

It typically takes a few days to have your first bowel movement after delivery. Your body went through a lot. Abdominal surgeries freak out your bowels a bit, so it will likely take longer for the first poop to arrive if you had a C-section. A lot of my patients are worried to tell me they haven't had a bowel movement yet when we talk about going home from the hospital. This is normal. In most cases, if you are at least passing gas and otherwise doing well, getting out of the hospital is not dependent on your ability to poop. If you do poop before going home, your health care team might appear weirdly happy for you.

No matter how you delivered, pooping will strain your most uncomfortable area. If you delivered vaginally, you likely have some swelling and stitches that will be impacted. If you had a C-section, the abdominal pressure you need in order to push for a bowel movement places stress on your incision.

Probably don't attempt your first poop while you're in a public restroom or while you have visitors. You're going to be in there a while, most likely crying. Take some pain medication and let it kick in before you go for it.

> Probably don't attempt your first poop while you're in a public restroom or while you have visitors.

As you might imagine, pooping will be more uncomfortable if you are constipated, just like it hurts more to get hit with a rock than a ball of Play-Doh. Poor hydration, low fiber intake, and use of narcotic medications can increase your risk of constipation. Drink lots of water, especially if you are breast- or chestfeeding, and eat fiber-rich foods. Manage your pain, but don't take narcotic medications if you don't need them.

Even for those who try to optimize the situation,

constipation is common postpartum. Use of a stool softener or laxative can be beneficial. Often, you are given (or at least have available) medications for this during your postpartum hospital stay. Ask if you can have a prescription for home. Otherwise, you can purchase something over the counter. Start by taking this daily for the first week if you need and can tolerate it, especially if you had a C-section, then see what you need from there. If these measures aren't helpful, try a suppository or enema (both can be found at any pharmacy).

One phoenix had an acquaintance with a poor postpartum pooping problem. That friend had refused to take laxatives and wasn't stringent with hydration postpartum, so she became constipated enough to tear her vaginal stitches the first couple times she had a post-delivery bowel movement. Knowing her friend's experience, that phoenix planned to use a stool softener, including a weaning schedule, and did not experience any issues.

> Constipation is common postpartum.

CONSTIPATION MEDICATIONS

- **Bulk-forming laxatives (Metamucil, Citrucel)** bulk up the stool to increase intestinal movement.

- **Enemas (Fleet Enema, mineral oil enema, saline enema)** expand the intestinal tract and stimulate motility.

- **Osmotic laxatives (MiraLAX, GoLYTELY)** increase water in intestines.

- **Saline laxatives (Milk of Magnesia, magnesium citrate)** increase water in intestines.

- **Stimulant laxatives (Senna, Dulcolax)** stimulate intestinal motility.

- **Stool softeners (Colace)** keep the stool soft so it is easier to pass.

- **Suppositories (Docusate, Bisacodyl)** are rectally administered medications that soften and hydrate stool.

In some circumstances, manual disimpaction is necessary. That's exactly what it sounds like: placing your or someone you trust's fingers (gloved and lubed, please, for everyone's sake) within your rectum to remove hard stool. If this is required, phoenixes typically see a health care professional rather than trying it at home.

If you are following these measures without any success, or if you are having severe abdominal pain associated with your constipation, not passing gas, experiencing nausea and vomiting, or consistently seeing blood in your bowel movements, you need to see a medical professional.

Pooping will get easier with time. Once you pass your first bowel movement, it won't be so scary.

WARNINGS

- Blood in stool

- Lack of bowel movements

- Not passing gas

- Persistent nausea and vomiting

- Severe abdominal pain

QUESTIONS

- Should I take a stool softener?

- What should I do if I'm taking a stool softener and it's not helping?

SUPPLIES

- Fiber-rich snacks

- Stool softener

- Water

> *Hemorrhoids in pregnancy . . . damn kids.*

Lisa, Minnesota

7

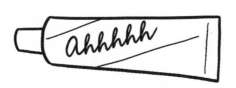

PAIN IN THE BUTT

Hemorrhoids

HOW CAN THINGS get any more glamorous? In pregnancy and postpartum, you may suffer from hemorrhoids.

Hemorrhoids are swollen vessels of the rectum (the bottom of your GI tract). They can be both external (on the outside of your anus, where you can see them) and internal (hiding up inside, where you can only feel their symptoms). Hemorrhoids can lead to significant discomfort and itching, and may cause bleeding with bowel movements. The general public seems to think hemorrhoids can't affect young people, but they can happen to almost anyone with a rectum — sorry to burst your bubble. They are more common in people who have had bad constipation or who pushed for long periods prior to delivery, but they also occur as a result of normal physiologic changes in pregnancy and postpartum.

Many phoenixes come to me worried that they have hemorrhoids based on something they saw with a mirror or felt with their hands, noting that they haven't had any symptoms. Sometimes I can confirm that hemorrhoids are present, and sometimes their exam doesn't reveal anything significant — but in all of these cases, I tell them they don't necessarily need to do anything differently because the hemorrhoids that may or may not exist aren't causing any problems.

Typically, hemorrhoids resolve on their own within the first couple weeks after delivery. Often, management strategies for vaginal delivery tearing are helpful for hemorrhoids that are causing symptoms: take ibuprofen or acetaminophen (please follow dosing instructions on the packaging, and make sure you don't have any contraindications to these medications), use your squirt bottle after going to the bathroom, apply soothing pads, sit on a cushion or pillow, avoid sitting for long periods, have a sitz bath. Over-the-counter topical creams (such as Preparation H) can ease the discomfort. Your health care clinician can prescribe a topical anesthetic if needed.

It is important to keep your stools soft to avoid straining with bowel movements. The more you put pressure on your rectum, the worse the hemorrhoids will get. Drink lots of water, increase fiber in your diet, and take a stool softener or laxative if needed.

> Typically, hemorrhoids resolve on their own within the first couple weeks after delivery.

Spots of blood may be occasionally noted after straining for a bowel movement due to hemorrhoid irritation. If you have persistent rectal bleeding with bowel movements or at any other time, you need to be evaluated by a medical professional. This could be a sign of something more worrisome.

Sometimes hemorrhoids clot off; these are referred to as thrombosed hemorrhoids. Signs include sudden severe rectal pain, persistent rectal bleeding, a darker (blue, purple, or even black) appearance of the hemorrhoid, or the hemorrhoid feeling hard to the touch. Your body will ultimately resorb the clot, but the pain and bleeding can be terrible for a couple days. You likely will not want to tackle this alone and should make an appointment at your medical clinician's office for evaluation.

If your hemorrhoids don't resolve or the symptoms aren't manageable, you may require a surgical procedure. This is not a surgery that your general OB/GYN clinician can perform (nor would you want them to), but they should be able to help you find the right specialist who can.

WARNINGS

- Blood in stools

- Dark tissue around the rectum

- Severe rectal pain

QUESTIONS

- Do I have hemorrhoids?

- How should I care for my hemorrhoids?

- Is surgery needed for my hemorrhoids?

SUPPLIES

- Fiber-rich snacks

- Hemorrhoid cream

- Ice packs

- Pillow

- Spray bottle

- Stool softener

- Tucks pads

- Water

KEGELS, KEGELS, KEGELS at every point in a woman's life. Talk about it early and often. No one ever explained it or showed me how until it went on so long that I needed physical therapy.

Kim, Delaware

8

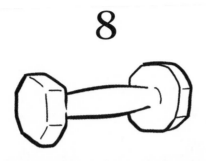

WORKING ON MY FITNESS

Exercise

WITH ALL THE free time you have (sorry, I shouldn't joke about that), you will want to work some physical activity into your schedule. If you had an uncomplicated pregnancy and vaginal delivery, you shouldn't have restrictions on your postpartum activity (besides sex, which we will talk about in chapter 10). I've had many phoenixes who had straightforward vaginal deliveries come back to my office for a routine postpartum appointment around six weeks and ask, "Can I start exercising now?" Yes, please! Go back to the past and do it also! If you had complications with your pregnancy or vaginal delivery, or if you delivered via C-section, talk to your delivery clinician about specific recommendations regarding timing and restrictions of resuming exercise. It may not be safe for you to work out right away.

> If you had an uncomplicated pregnancy and vaginal delivery, you shouldn't have restrictions on your postpartum activity.

Whatever your favorite form of exercise is, once you've received the okay from a medical professional, ease back into it slowly. Even if you were able to exercise well all the way through pregnancy, delivery itself and your body's need to recover will probably set you back a bit. If you're a long-distance runner, start with shorter runs. If you're a weight lifter, back off on the weights you're using. If you were a champ at your CrossFit gym, plan on being a mediocre participant.

If you haven't ever really had an exercise routine, now is a great time to establish one. Don't push yourself too hard, but do get yourself moving. If all you can manage is a short walk every day, that's better than nothing. Your journey as a phoenix may bring you to better health.

After a baby grew inside you, some of your muscles, ligaments, and joints may be a little . . . shot. Due to the pressure of the pregnancy and the stretching to accommodate it, your pelvis, abdomen, and back are likely in need of some attention. Pelvic floor relaxation, diastasis recti (the separation of the abdominal muscles), and any disruption to the biomechanical ical aspects that allow your body to optimally function can lead to chronic pelvic pain, pain with intercourse, difficulties with bowel movements or urination, poor posture, abdominal pain, lower back pain, or hernias.

> Don't push yourself too hard, but do get yourself moving.

One phoenix experienced abdominal pains and sensations that were hard to describe after delivery. It took weeks and multiple visits with a handful of doctors for her to receive the diagnosis of diastasis recti, and she wasn't provided any recommendations for how to manage it once it was identified. She searched online on her own for appropriate physical therapy resources.

Directed exercises can improve these muscle-related issues. Incorporate into your routine exercises to strengthen your pelvic floor and abdominal muscles. Think about Kegel exercises, squats, wall sits, cat/cow pose (put yourself in a tabletop position on all fours, then curl your back up and down), pelvic lifts (lie down on your back with your legs bent up and slowly raise and lower your bottom), and abdominal compressions (clench your abs while imagining raising your belly button up toward your head on a string). Try to avoid sit-ups, crunches, or planks – these simply increase pressure in your abdomen and can worsen diastasis.

Not all phoenixes can tackle these issues alone, and you shouldn't have to. Many physical therapists, yogis, osteopaths, chiropractors, and massage therapists specialize in postpartum care and/or pelvic floor issues. Ask your obstetrics clinician for a referral to someone they trust who provides quality care related to these concerns.

EXERCISES

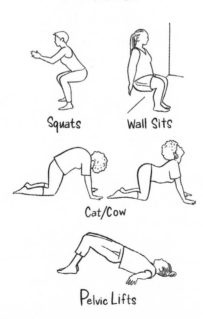

Squats   Wall Sits

Cat/Cow

Pelvic Lifts

Some exercise classes directed to phoenixes are offered by gyms or online. If you're a member of a gym, see if it has any recommendations. Many online programs come with a cost, and if you pursue one, look at reviews and carefully consider what you are getting for your money. YouTube has plenty of free videos as well.

WARNINGS

- Persistent pain with exercise

- Persistent shortness of breath during exercise

QUESTIONS

- Do you have recommendations for a pelvic floor physical therapist?

- What activity restrictions do I have?

- What exercises would be good for me?

SUPPLIES

- A comfortable and supportive sports bra

- Comfortable exercise clothing

- Gym membership or home exercise equipment (even if that's just walking shoes!)

- Water

Dear lord, the night sweating. Nothing helped. I just wish I had been warned about it! I did a ton of reading on what to expect, but never saw it mentioned until I searched it specifically. For me, it was a solid eight weeks of soaking wet sheets, then another month or so of tapering off. Both pregnancies.

Nikki, Minnesota

9

YOUR BODY IS A WONDERLAND

Body Changes

YOUR BODY IS a wonderland — as in *Alice in Wonderland*, where things can grow and shrink and become curiouser and curiouser.

Your weight has changed, and it might be concentrated in new areas. For some phoenixes, everything eventually settles back to normal. Others need to adjust to a new normal. Keep at least some of your old wardrobe on hand just in case, but make sure you have items that fit comfortably through your transitions.

Your feet have probably grown, and some of your favorite shoes might not fit anymore. Some phoenixes go up a full shoe size with each pregnancy without ever having their feet go back to the way they were. If you have a closet full of beloved shoes that now don't fit, give them one last hug and bring them to a donation center for a new owner to love.

> For some phoenixes, everything eventually settles back to normal. Others need to adjust to a new normal.

Your nose and ears may be bigger as well (all the better to smell and hear you with, my dear). It won't be as dramatic as, say, an elderly man compared to his younger self, but you may notice a subtle difference as you examine yourself in the mirror.

Abdominal binders can help with abdominal, pelvic, and hip discomfort as your body adjusts back to its prepregnancy state. Some phoenixes simply feel more confident with a binder or shapewear as well (but you don't have to use these products if you don't want to).

Wear appropriately fitted and well-supportive bras or tops as your chest size fluctuates during this time. Most lingerie stores do bra fittings for free. Your bra size may be forever changed! This is true for both the cups and the band, as many phoenixes' ribcages permanently widen after pregnancy.

Your eyesight may be blurrier and it may be more difficult to focus your gaze. This is likely to improve, typically within a few months. This change often stems from hormonal effects and fluid retention. Of course, make sure you can see well enough to navigate life safely, but maybe opt for a cheap, less-fashionable pair of specs during this time if needed, rather than breaking the bank on expensive new glasses. If your eyesight hasn't improved by a few months postpartum or is significantly impairing your function, see your eye doctor. If you're seeing flashes or spots in your vision, this is not normal and requires evaluation.

Hot flashes, night sweats, and cold sweats are common. These are a result of the normal hormonal fluctuations in the postpartum period in addition to your body's need to remove previously retained fluid. Wear layers and have a change of clothes ready next to your bed at nighttime.

Your hair is going to fall out. This can be especially traumatizing to some. You have likely become accustomed to having shiny, thick locks in pregnancy, but they will disappear in chunks. Hormonal changes affect normal cycles of hair growth and loss while you're pregnant, causing hair to spend more time on your head. When hormones again change postpartum, all that extra hair comes out. A friend described seeing a small toupee collecting in the shower drain every morning. Continuing to take vitamins, avoiding heat treatments, limiting shampooing, and using a gentle brush or comb can be helpful, but nothing can truly stop this process. Many phoenixes tell me something must be wrong due to all the hair they are losing. Let it go.

Your hair texture might also change. Phoenixes report their locks going from wavy to straight and vice versa. A new hair routine might be in your future!

> You have likely become accustomed to having shiny, thick locks in pregnancy, but they will disappear in chunks.

Your skin is likely left with stretch marks, and some might be permanent. You may be able to reduce their appearance, if desired, by staying hydrated, moisturizing frequently, and exercising. Some phoenixes are predisposed to having more dramatic skin changes in pregnancy and postpartum.

Your body might be different now, but it brought you through pregnancy and delivery. Show it some love.

WARNINGS

- Chest pain

- Extreme fatigue not improved with rest

- Funny heartbeats

- Inability to lose weight with a routine of healthy diet and exercise

- Persistent pain not improved with medications

- Shortness of breath, especially at rest

- Significant swelling that does not improve with time

- Skin changes that are itchy or painful

- Spots, flashes, or blind areas in your visual field

QUESTIONS

- Are the changes I'm noticing normal (mention anything different that's happening so it can all be taken into consideration together)?

- Do I need an eye exam?

- Do you recommend any lab testing?

- Should I use an abdominal binder?

SUPPLIES

- Abdominal binder

- Appropriately fitting clothes and shoes

We tried to have sex and it didn't feel quite right. It freaked me out, so we haven't tried again.

Anonymous

10

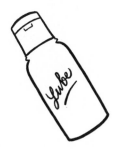

LET'S GET IT ON

Sex

IMMEDIATELY AFTER DELIVERY, most phoenixes think, "I will never have sex again!" For a small subset, this may turn out to be true. You'd be surprised, though, how quickly some people remember that they enjoy sex.

Universally, it is recommended to avoid penetrative intercourse (this includes body parts or sex toys inserted vaginally or rectally) for at least the first six weeks postpartum. Your reproductive organs need time to heal and don't need any prodding. Don't let anyone — including the little devil on your shoulder — talk you into intercourse prior to this. Foreplay and external sexual activities can also be uncomfortable during this time due to nipple sensitivity, uterine contractions, vulvar swelling, and other changes.

> Your reproductive organs need time to heal and don't need any prodding.

Please consider the location of any stitches if you or your partner(s) attempt any stimulation — let those places heal before you use them for fun!

Many phoenixes struggle with feeling sexy after delivery. Your body has changed, and you might not be comfortable with those changes. Don't feel obligated to put a ton of effort into it, but wearing an outfit that has always made you feel hot, playing your favorite jams, pampering yourself a bit, and remembering that your partner(s) WANTS YOU can help you get your groove back.

Your body's changes and how you feel about them, in addition to the fact that a lot of your brainpower may be focused on a new tiny human or the absence thereof, can really minimize your libido. There's unfortunately no magic cure for libido changes. Do not force sex if you're not feeling it. You can be intimate with your partner(s) (or yourself) in other ways.

Your first go at any sexual activity after delivery is

unlikely to be your best work. You're going to need to ease into it and go slowly. Communicate clearly with your partner what feels good and what really doesn't.

If it's too uncomfortable, it's okay to stop. Don't get frustrated. Many phoenixes have told me they tried to have sex once and then took months to attempt it again because of discomfort. If at first you don't

> Do not force sex if you're not feeling it.

succeed, try, try again! It can take weeks or months for sex to be free of some discomfort (not *pain*) or awkwardness after delivery. This is especially the case for penetrative intercourse but can be true for many sexual activities.

You may notice milk leakage with sexual contact, particularly nipple stimulation. It is probably best to warn your partner(s) about this. Roll with it.

For penetrative sexual activity, use lube (silicone-based lubricants tend to work better than water-based ones, as they don't dry out as quickly; coconut or olive oil is a good approach for those sensitive to additives in commercial lubricants). You will likely have more vaginal dryness than usual, especially if lactating, and lube will improve that. USE A LOT OF LUBE! Buy all the lube you can. Prepare more lube than you've ever used before, and then double that.

You really can't overdo it on the lube. Did I mention lube?

It's not unusual for sex to feel different forever —

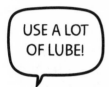

but different doesn't mean bad. Your body isn't the same as it once was, and that's okay. Sensations might have changed from what you've experienced in the past.

Repeat after me: sex should not hurt. (There's a caveat for well-communicated, mutually agreed-upon, purposefully inflicted pain for pleasure.) If you experience persistent pain anywhere with sexual activity, talk to your gynecologist. Pelvic floor physical therapy, surgical revision of poorly healed tearing, infection treatment, estrogen cream, breast or chest imaging, hemorrhoid treatment, or colonoscopy may be recommended.

Lube.

WARNINGS

- Abnormal vaginal discharge
- Bleeding after sex
- Persistent pain with sex

QUESTIONS

- Is what I'm feeling during sex normal?
- When can I start having intercourse again?
- When can I start sexual activity again?
- Which lubricants do you recommend?

SUPPLIES

- Lube

*I never want to
do this again.*

Anonymous

11

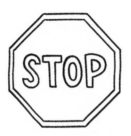

STOP IN THE NAME OF LOVE

Birth Control

SOME PHOENIXES OVULATE within six weeks of delivery, and often your first ovulation will occur before your first period. This means you can become pregnant again a lot sooner than most people think. This sometimes leads to surprises.

Whether or not you're planning to be pregnant again, if you plan to have vaginal intercourse with a semen-producing partner, you should be thinking about birth control. Pregnancies that occur in close succession carry an increased risk of maternal anemia (low number of red blood cells), preterm labor, and babies that grow small. Phoenixes who have a C-section and then have another pregnancy soon after have an increased risk of the incision on the uterus coming open, an issue called uterine rupture, which is dangerous to the phoenix and the baby. In general, at least eighteen months between delivery and conception is recommended for phoenixes under thirty-five, or twelve months for phoenixes older than thirty-five (balancing other risks that increase at that time).

> You can become pregnant again a lot sooner than most people think.

If you required medications to help you conceive or went through in-vitro fertilization, this does not necessarily mean you cannot conceive without these measures in the future. A surprising number of phoenixes do. I've worked with patients who felt they didn't need contraception due to their history of reproductive assistance and quickly ended up spontaneously pregnant in the postpartum period. This often creates a difficult and emotional situation. Even if another pregnancy eventually would be happy news, to ensure the best outcomes for everyone, phoenixes who have utilized reproductive assistance and plan penis-in-vagina sex should still use birth control.

Many birth control methods also have noncontraceptive benefits, such as controlling acne, physical and mental symptoms surrounding menses, very heavy and/or painful periods, endometriosis, fibroids, and conditions that cause abnormalities in ovulation and menstruation. Some contraceptive methods also reduce the risk of certain cancers. You don't have to be having sex at all to want or need "birth" control.

CONTRACEPTIVES

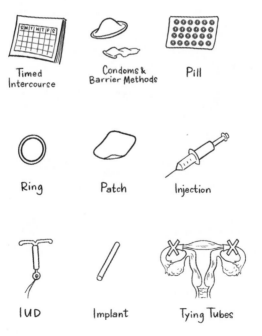

Timed Intercourse

Condoms & Barrier Methods

Pill

Ring

Patch

Injection

IUD

Implant

Tying Tubes

Abstinence is the only 100-percent effective form of birth control. This is not desirable for many phoenixes, although it may be for a while after delivery. At least six weeks without intercourse is recommended postpartum.

Consistent lactation generally delays the resumption of menstrual cycles (this is called lactational amenorrhea), but this isn't a surefire way to prevent pregnancy. You might know someone who is still breast- or chestfeeding their newborn but is already pregnant again, which may or may not have been planned.

> Abstinence is the only 100-percent effective from of birth control. This is not desirable for many phoenixes.

Some people are great at natural family planning or timed intercourse — essentially avoiding intercourse during the time surrounding ovulation when conception is most likely to occur. In a standard twenty-eight-day menstrual cycle with the first day of bleeding as day one, ovulation generally occurs right in the middle, around day fourteen or fifteen. For longer or shorter cycles, this is not the case. For longer cycles, ovulation is instead tracked in a retrospective manner, as it most likely occurs around fourteen days prior to the subsequent period. For shorter cycles, it sometimes follows the approximately fourteen-day rule, but the interval may be shorter. This means you have to understand your cycles over time to predict ovulation using a calendar alone. Monitoring cervical mucus, which becomes more of an egg-white consistency during ovulation, or basal body temperature, which rises slightly just after ovulation, can help identify this timing as well. After ejaculation, sperm can live inside the vagina and reproductive tract for up to five days. After the physical release of the egg, the egg and sperm can still meet up for up to another day. Appropriately avoiding intercourse at the correct times can be hard for some people and can be an unreliable method for phoenixes who have irregular periods.

Condoms and other barrier methods — when used consistently and correctly with every act of intercourse — can be very effective. Unfortunately, human error means many people don't use them consistently or correctly with every act (overlooking expiration dates, wearing two condoms at once, buying the wrong size condoms while thinking they are totally the right size, putting the condom on too late, taking the condom off too soon, deciding "Hey, it's just this once without a condom, what could go wrong?" etc.), and they end up not being optimal. Internal condoms that are placed in the vagina also exist but are not as widely available, and they often oddly require a prescription. Don't forget: always use some type of condom to protect against sexually transmitted infections if you have a new partner, multiple partners, or partners who have other partners. Other barrier methods include diaphragms, cervical caps, or contraceptive sponges. These methods are physical blocks that prevent the sperm from getting up to the egg. They are sometimes used in conjunction with spermicide, a chemical product that kills sperm.

> Don't forget: always use some type of condom to protect against sexually transmitted infections.

Caution needs to be taken with the initiation of estrogen-containing contraceptives (such as the patch, the ring, and some pills) too soon after delivery. The heightened risk of blood clots in your extremities or lungs that exists throughout pregnancy continues postpartum. It is highest throughout the first three weeks and continues until six to twelve weeks postpartum. Taking estrogen-containing medications during that time further increases your risk of a blood clot, which in some circumstances is life-threatening. Estrogen-containing medications can also impact lactation and should not be started before a good routine has been established for those who wish to breast- or chestfeed. Most estrogen-containing methods are intended to be prescribed in a manner that allows a monthly break for menses during which the method isn't used. If you've taken pills before, the sugar pills (placebos) at the end of a pill pack are simply there to help keep you on track during that off week. Using estrogen-containing methods back-to-back (skipping the placebo/off week and going right into the next pack, patch, or ring) can suppress menstruation (this is safe when medically induced) and increase contraceptive efficacy.

Progesterone-only contraceptives do not appear to carry the adverse effects of estrogen-containing methods and can theoretically be initiated at any time postpartum. Check with your prenatal care clinician to find out when you can practically start them. With pills that contain only progesterone, it is important to take them as close as possible to the same time every day, as they have less wiggle room than standard pills that contain both estrogen and progesterone. It can be difficult to stick to taking a medication at the same time every day in general, and especially so when you are dealing with the physical, mental, emotional, and scheduling changes of the postpartum period. The birth control shot (injected every three months), subdermal (under the skin of the upper arm) contraceptive implant (lasts three years), and hormonal intrauterine devices (IUDs, good for three to six years, depending on which one you choose) all only contain types of progesterone. Any progesterone-only medication can cause some irregular bleeding, and some phoenixes have no periods long-term while using progesterone-only methods.

All hormonal forms of contraception have the potential to lessen the bleeding, pain, and other symptoms associated with periods. Potential side effects from hormonal forms of birth control in general may include weight gain, changes to mental health, headaches, nausea and vomiting, and breast or chest tenderness. Is there anything else you've experienced that caused these symptoms? I don't know, maybe something that made you read this book in the first place? The symptoms of pregnancy are generally much more significant than the side effects of birth control. Consider which would be more optimal for you.

The copper IUD contains no hormones and lasts for ten years. It does not impact the timing of periods; in some cases, it makes periods crampier and heavier. Rarely are patients unable to use this type of IUD due to its copper content.

In some delivery centers, either type of IUD or

the subdermal contraceptive implant can be placed immediately after delivery. This is an excellent choice if you are hoping for long-term, very effective, reversible contraception, especially if you may have issues with following up with a health care clinician postpartum. Check if this would be a possibility for you.

For those who are sure they are done with childbearing, sterilization is an option. Most people refer to this as tying tubes. A portion of the fallopian tube (the path the egg takes after ovulation to enter the uterus) on each side may be removed or constricted, or the tubes may be removed completely. This can be performed immediately postpartum at the time of a C-section or through a small incision under the belly button soon after vaginal delivery. Tubal surgery can also be performed later on through a laparoscopic approach (small incisions in the abdomen with the use of a camera). Across all types of available sterilization, regardless of one's sex, vasectomy of a semen-producing partner is the most effective, least invasive form.

> No one method of birth control is perfect for everyone.

Notably, the subdermal contraceptive implant and both types of IUDs are just as — if not more — effective in preventing pregnancy than tubal surgery.

Again, no method besides abstinence is 100-percent effective, and all these contraceptive methods come with a small chance of pregnancy.

No one method of birth control is perfect for everyone. All types come with pros and cons, and every phoenix's body uniquely responds to contraceptive methods. Talk to your prenatal care clinician about what might work best for you so you have a plan in place when it's time to get down again (and/or if you want to use prescription birth control for other purposes).

WARNINGS

- Bleeding through more than one pad per hour persistently

- Chest pain

- Negative mood changes

- Painful swelling in a leg or arm

- Shortness of breath

- Vaginal irritation or pain after condom use

QUESTIONS

- How should I best plan for future pregnancies?

- How should I best plan for never becoming pregnant again?

- Is there any type of birth control I shouldn't use?

- What types of birth control would you recommend for my circumstances?

Breastfeeding is hard. I wish I knew a lot of things. Even though your kid is sucking on the breast, they aren't always eating. I was freaking out for a while about how much she was eating and her weight gain, so once she was able to stay awake long enough to suck properly, I'd let her suck for over an hour at a time. That significantly cut down on my sleep, and then I discovered she wasn't swallowing for a lot of that time, and I could cut down on it somewhat. Even when we got the hang of breastfeeding, it waxes and wanes how well we do. We've gone for stretches of weeks where things are a struggle again, but we just keep trying to get back into a rhythm.

Margo, Texas

I had pain with breastfeeding up until eleven weeks postpartum. I saw a lactation consultant probably eight to ten times. I developed clogged ducts every week, going back to work with the stress, getting into a rhythm with pumping. Sunflower lecithin has been a great daily supplement to help emulsify the fat. I also tried six sessions of cold laser therapy at a chiropractic clinic, along with frequent emptying of the breasts and trying to remain stress free (not that easy)! I think some people are just more susceptible to clogs, and I definitely am. But it's been almost seven months and my supply is still good, so I am happy to keep going!

Britta, Minnesota

12

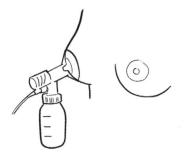

MILK IT FOR ALL IT'S WORTH

Breast- or Chestfeeding

THERE'S NO USE crying over spilled milk. Say this to a breast- or chestfeeding phoenix if you'd like to be punched in the face.

Feeding a baby your own human milk has many benefits. It boosts the baby's immune system to reduce risks of multiple types of infections (respiratory, urinary tract, gastrointestinal, ear, blood). Babies experience fewer digestive problems and have a lower risk of later developing diabetes, lymphoma, leukemia, and childhood obesity. It can help with postpartum weight loss and decrease the risk of the phoenix later developing breast or ovarian cancer.

There are a few medical contraindications to feeding a baby your own human milk. Talk to your prenatal care clinician about your circumstances.

Most phoenixes are encouraged to try breast- or chestfeeding. However, it can be hard — really, really, really hard. When I ask phoenixes about their postpartum struggles, this is without a doubt the biggest area that causes distress. Many tell me they didn't realize how difficult and defeating it would be.

Although medical groups promote the process, society creates obstacles for it. Phoenixes are made to feel that they need to hide in uncomfortable places so that no one harasses them for exposing body parts that might otherwise be covered. Some areas ridiculously impose legal ramifications for public nipple exposure in the setting of feeding a baby. Not only does this stigmatize and obstruct the process, but because of this pressure for secrecy, most phoenixes have never seen breast- or chestfeeding in person before and thus do not know how it looks when done correctly. Many phoenixes feel strong expectations to go back to work sooner than they would like, and a lot of them do not have jobs that provide adequate time, space, and resources for pumping or bringing a baby to work.

Start preparing for feeding your baby as soon as you can. Lactation classes and support groups are offered at a cost or for free in many communities. Look into La Leche League to help identify these resources in your community. Talk to people in your life who have fed from the chest to gain their insight. Read about breast- or chestfeeding in books or online; www.kellymom.com is a convenient resource with tons of information. Watch YouTube videos to see what a proper latch looks like; "Dr. Jack Newman's Visual Guide to Breastfeeding" is an incredibly helpful thirty-minute video. Check with your insurance company regarding pump coverage requirements so you can obtain one well in advance. Talk to your partner or other support person to make a plan for sharing feeding duties with pumped milk. Start making a plan about when, where, and how you will pump at your workplace. Buy nipple shields (regular, gel, silver — all kinds!) and nipple cream. If you are a gestational carrier or placing the baby for adoption, consider the potential for you to donate milk to the family for a while.

Although medical groups promote breast- or chest-feeding, society creates obstacles for it.

If you plan to breast- or chestfeed, insist on at least

one hour of immediate skin-to-skin contact with the baby after delivery, as long as it is medically safe to do this. Start attempting feeding as soon as you can. Ask every nurse who enters your postpartum room for tips. Feed the baby frequently (every two to three hours) and on demand for the first few days.

Initially, your milk ducts produce colostrum, a more concentrated fluid that is rich in protein and antibodies. You might not produce a lot of fluid right away, but the baby is still likely getting enough nutrition due to the makeup of colostrum. Your milk will usually come in within two to four days after delivery.

Ensuring the appropriate latch is hard. Make sure a knowledgeable nurse or lactation consultant watches you feed the baby at your chest and/or pump before you leave the hospital. A large portion of your areola — not just the nipple itself — should be in the baby's mouth. The baby's lips should be flanged out. The baby's chin should slightly dig into your chest tissue. There should be space, however, between the baby's nose and your skin.

You will not always hear your baby swallow, but you might. If you watch the baby's face, you should be able to see repetitive, large sucking motions with intermittent pauses that allow for swallowing.

If the baby seems to be dozing off, or just nibbling

A GOOD LATCH

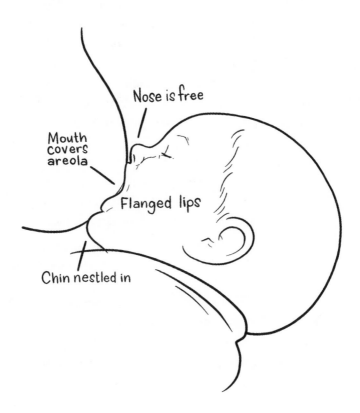

Nose is free

Mouth covers areola

Flanged lips

Chin nestled in

and not actually feeding, apply some compression to your breast or chest (act like you're squeezing a water bottle) or switch to the other side.

Breast- or chestfeeding will be uncomfortable, but it generally shouldn't be painful. Your areolae and nipples may be sore, but they shouldn't bleed. Severe pain and bleeding may be a sign of an inappropriate latch. Nipple creams and pads can help with discomfort and dryness. Some phoenixes find pain relief and assistance with tissue repair via low-level laser therapy that can be accessed at specialty clinics. If you have persistent issues, talk to a lactation consultant, pediatrician, or obstetrics clinician to work on technique.

Monitoring the baby's weight (performed at the pediatrician's office) and wet diapers (tallied by you) can help ensure the baby is getting enough milk. There should be multiple wet diapers each day. If the baby isn't making wet diapers, contact your pediatrician.

Do not allow your milk to get backed up and overfill. Called engorgement, this can be incredibly painful for you. If this seems to be happening, apply warm compresses, take ibuprofen or acetaminophen (please follow dosing instructions on the packaging and make sure you don't have any contraindications to these medications), and express milk between feedings.

Sometimes you may end up with a clogged milk duct, which will feel like a tender lump. This can be treated the same way as engorgement. Taking a supplement of sunflower lecithin can help reduce your milk's thickness and prevent the recurrence of clogged ducts.

If your chest feels hot to the touch, appears red, and is in pain, you may have an infection called mastitis. A common reaction is to stop feeding or pumping from the affected side. DO NOT DO THIS. This can cause the infection to build up and create a pocket of infected fluid and tissue called an abscess. Let the milk flow; it's also safe to feed it to the baby. Call your obstetrics clinician, as you will likely need antibiotics to clear the infection. Sometimes a procedure to drain an abscess is required.

One phoenix had never heard of clogged ducts, so she didn't know what to monitor. She noticed a lumpy area in one breast with reduced milk flow from that side. She decided to reduce feeding and pumping from that side and increase it with the other breast. After the clogged duct persisted, she developed a severe case of mastitis that worsened her sleep deprivation, contributed to PTSD, and nearly landed her in the hospital. Don't overlook lumps, bumps, pain, skin changes, or the appearance of any fluid that doesn't look like milk coming from the nipple.

You are likely to leak milk, often at inopportune times. Your body will start to adapt to cues, so simply hearing a baby cry or someone inadvertently brushing up against your chest may stimulate milk letdown. Be prepared for this when you're out and about.

Freshly pumped milk is safe for consumption for up to four hours at room temperature. It can be stored in a refrigerator for three to five days or in a freezer for up to one year. If you store too much, you can donate milk to local milk banks for other parents to use. Conversely, you can obtain milk from local milk banks if you want to provide your baby with human milk but are unable to provide your own.

> You are likely to leak milk, often at inopportune times.

Fenugreek is an herb popularly used in capsule form or in tea to increase milk supply. It is safe to use, though results vary. Increasing your frequency of breast- or chestfeeding and pumping increases your supply as well.

Make sure to stay adequately hydrated! Producing milk literally drains you. Drink at least a gallon of water daily if you can. This will help you feel physically better overall and help you maintain your supply.

Emotions and lactation go hand in hand. Emotions fluctuate a lot postpartum, a variability that can last throughout the time you breast- or chestfeed. Some phoenixes experience dysphoric milk ejection reflex, in which they experience negative feelings accompanying milk letdown that often last a few minutes.

> Emotions and lactation go hand in hand.

It is okay to supplement with formula or switch to it completely if needed or desired. If feeding the baby your own human milk doesn't work out for any reason, *you are not a failure*. Your worth as a caregiver and a human is not related to milk production. Sometimes babies don't obtain the nutrition they need because phoenixes become too obsessive about strictly breast- or chestfeeding. Making sure the baby is sufficiently fed is far better than avoiding supplementation.

Give yourself some grace. There is a lot of pressure and demand with trying to satisfy your personal goals. Do your best.

WARNINGS

- Bleeding nipples

- Breast or chest lump

- Discolored nipple discharge

- Fevers and chills

- Inability to produce any fluid from a nipple

- Persistent, severe breast or chest pain

- Redness of the breast or chest

- Shooting nipple pain

QUESTIONS

- Am I doing this right?

- Are the changes I've noticed to my breast or chest tissue normal?

- Should I be concerned about clogged ducts or mastitis?

- Should I be supplementing?

- What can I do to increase supply?

- What community resources can help me with breast- or chestfeeding?

- What should I do if I think I have clogged ducts or mastitis?

SUPPLIES

- Breast or chest pump

- Bottle brush

- Bottle drying rack

- Bottles and nipples

- Fenugreek supplements

- Nipple cream

- Nipple shields

- Sunflower lecithin

I was told to wrap ACE bandages around my chest tightly. This caused me severe pain and led to an infection, which made the experience after stillbirth even more difficult.

Anonymous

13

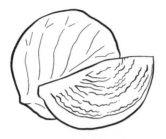

NOT GONNA DO IT

NOT Breast- or Chestfeeding

NOT BREAST- OR chestfeeding is not necessarily synonymous with formula-feeding, but it can be. Phoenixes who experience a stillbirth or deliver a baby who has other parents may decide they want to prevent lactation as much as possible. Some phoenixes who plan on formula-feeding have the same desire. There's no surefire way to prevent any milk flow at all, but some measures can help.

Wear a well-fitted, supportive bra or top. This does not mean tightly binding your chest in a painful and restrictive manner, which can actually worsen pain and milk leakage. If you typically wear a binder on your chest, take a break from this for a few weeks. Make sure your bras and tops are comfortable and not too tight or loose. Sports bras can be particularly helpful.

Avoid nipple stimulation as much as possible. Even hot water in the shower can cause stimulation, so don't rely on this tempting measure for comfort.

Placing cold compresses in your bra can help with discomfort and can reduce milk production. You might use a fancy wrapped gel pack from a pharmacy or a simple bag of peas from the freezer. Cold cabbage leaves placed within the bra and changed every two hours can potentially improve the discomfort of engorgement and reduce milk production.

There is limited, inconsistent evidence that herbs including sage, peppermint, chasteberry, parsley, and jasmine may reduce milk production. Consuming these is likely most tolerable in tea form.

Medications can be given in the hospital to prevent lactation, but their routine use has fallen out of favor due to the potential for significant side effects. Talk to your prenatal care and/or delivery clinician about your specific circumstances.

You are likely to still produce a little milk and may leak milk at unexpected times regardless of what you do to prevent it. You can hand-express small amounts of milk if you are too uncomfortable.

WARNINGS

- Breast or chest lump

- Discolored nipple discharge

- Fevers and chills

- Persistent, severe breast or chest pain

- Redness of the breast or chest

QUESTIONS

- Are the sensations I'm feeling in my breast or chest tissue normal?

- How can I best plan avoiding lactation?

SUPPLIES

- Cold cabbage leaves

- Cold compresses

- Well-fitted, supportive bra

> I wish my doctor had told me breastfeeding doesn't work for everyone. Don't spend your maternity leave worrying about how "breast is best." Do what works for you and baby, and enjoy the time off that you have with your newborn.

Erika, Minnesota

14

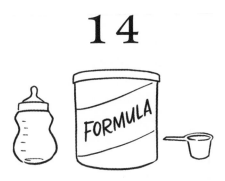

FORMULA FOR SUCCESS

Formula-Feeding

HUMAN MILK IS not the only way to feed a baby. Breast- or chestfeeding/pumping may be unadvised due to medical problems or required medications. Or it may be physically impractical or incompatible with good mental health. The baby might be separated from the phoenix. The phoenix may not want to breast- or chestfeed. It may simply not work.

These things are all okay, no matter how anyone else makes you feel about it.

In the four years of my OB/GYN residency, not once did I receive any education about formula-feeding.

Granted, our education regarding breast- or chest-feeding wasn't top notch either, but at least it existed. Formula-feeding was a topic to avoid and ignore. Many hospitals have Baby-Friendly certifications, which are an effort from the United Nations Children's Fund and the World Health Organization to ensure all maternity centers provide adequate lactation support. Again, feeding a baby human milk can be great and is encouraged in many circumstances, but I've noticed that the staunch emphasis on being Baby-Friendly often doesn't come across as very phoenix-friendly. Phoenixes who need or want to formula-feed for whatever reason end up feeling highly judged and stigmatized.

> I've noticed that the staunch emphasis on being Baby-Friendly often doesn't come across as very phoenix-friendly.

Some phoenixes who desire to breast- or chestfeed tell me they worry about encountering problems with it because they don't know the first thing about the alternative of formula-feeding. They are afraid to ask about formula-feeding because they don't want to be judged for using it, a big area in the ever-prevalent shame culture of parenting.

One phoenix told me formula was never mentioned across several prenatal classes, even when she specifically asked about it, and her obstetrician had no helpful advice for successful formula-feeding when she indicated she wasn't planning to breast-feed. The phoenix noted significant formula-feeding criticism in online parenting groups. Luckily, she found the Fed is Best group online, which helped identify resources and information. She was ultimately successful with safe formula-feeding, but she didn't expect or appreciate such a struggle.

Formula has its benefits, such as more accurate knowledge regarding the amount and nutritional content of what the baby is consuming. People other than the phoenix can be more involved in feeding and caring for the baby, an important consideration for many couples but one crucial for most adopted babies. The phoenix can better obtain the important rest needed to heal after delivery and to function as normally as possible. The phoenix has more flexibility in returning to work or other activities.

Of the many types of formula, choose one that is FDA-approved and iron-fortified. Other aspects — such as cow milk protein-based, soy-based, hydro-lyzed, hypoallergenic, powder, concentrated liquid, ready-to-use — may help you pick a formula based on your own preferences and the baby's tolerance. Find coupons for many popular brands of formula online;

because the internet knows everything about you, you've probably received them by e-mail already.

Always check the expiration date on any formula, and do not use any that is expired.

In addition to obtaining formula, you will need to have plenty of bottles and nipples on hand. There are lots of different types of these, and there is no best combination. Buy a couple kinds to start, then see what works best for you and the baby.

Sterilize all supplies prior to use, whether by boiling, steaming, or washing them in the dishwasher. Clean every item well between each use. You may choose to sterilize with each wash. It is recommended that you do this if your baby was born prematurely or has a compromised immune system. Many people find a bottle brush and a bottle drying rack to be handy.

Follow the instructions on the formula packaging for preparation, and add only the exact amount of water indicated. Too much or too little water can be harmful to the baby. If you are on a public water system, you can use tap water only if it has less than 0.7 mg/L fluoride — too much fluoride can harm the baby's teeth. Otherwise, purchase nonfluoridated water.

Stir and swirl to mix formula. Shaking creates bubbles that can give the baby more gas. Due to the way formula is digested, formula-fed babies tend to be gassier than those drinking human milk. You're going to need a lot of burp cloths!

If you choose to heat up the formula (you don't have to), do NOT heat it in the microwave. It heats unevenly and can make some parts dangerously hot. Instead, place the bottle with prepared formula inside of it in a bowl of hot water until a drop of the formula feels warm when squirted onto your skin.

For the first week, feed the baby every three to four hours with 1.5 to 2 oz. of formula. Feed on demand. For the first four to six months, offer the baby 2.5 oz. of formula per pound of body weight throughout the day. You can space the feedings more over time.

> If you choose to heat up the formula (you don't have to), do NOT heat it in the microwave.

It's always important to touch base with your pediatrician at each appointment to make sure no changes are necessary with the type, amount, and frequency of formula-feeding based on the baby's needs.

Refer to the Centers for Disease Control and Prevention (CDC) for additional information regarding safe formula-feeding. This was a primary source for my self-education on the topic.

WARNINGS

- Abnormal or no bowel movements from the baby

- Bloating of the baby's abdomen

- Extreme flatulence from the baby

- Lack of wet diapers

- Persistent vomiting from the baby

- The baby crying inconsolably

- Unexplained rashes on the baby's skin

QUESTIONS

- Am I doing this right?

- Are there community resources to help me with this?

- Do you have any formula samples or coupons, or know where I can get them?

- I've noticed [fill in the blank] after the baby drinks formula. Should I change types?

SUPPLIES

- Bottle brush

- Bottle drying rack

- Bottles and nipples

- Formula

- Formula coupons

- Nonfluoridated water

All I wanted after delivery was to eat a whole pizza! I made my husband get one delivered to the hospital.

Anonymous

15

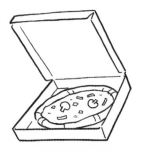

I CAN'T BELIEVE I ATE
THE WHOLE THING

Foods, Drinks, and Consumables

THROUGHOUT PREGNANCY, THERE'S a good chance your dietary habits modified at least somewhat. We always recommend avoiding or cautiously consuming certain types of fish, meats, and cheeses, for instance. We recommend safe amounts of caffeine, and we advise against alcohol in any amount. Persistent issues with nausea or reflux might have taken some of your favorite foods off the menu. You may have been watching your carb intake due to gestational diabetes. Now that the pregnancy is out of your belly, you're probably excited about some of the things you want to GET. IN. YOUR. BELLY. Bring on the buffet! Time to feast!

Okay, slow down there, buddy. Yes, take this opportunity to treat yourself and indulge a little, but don't go out of control. Just because you don't have to worry about the pregnancy anymore doesn't mean you don't have to worry about your own health or the exposures to the baby, if you're breast- or chestfeeding. You don't have to be a total health nut, and treats are okay in moderation, but you do need nourishment to heal and to support a healthy body and mind.

> Yes, take this opportunity to treat yourself and indulge a little, but don't go out of control.

As is the case for any time in your life, a healthy, balanced diet is important. Variety to the types of foods you eat not only keeps your meals exciting but provides the appropriate building blocks to keep your body running. The United States Department of Agriculture has backed away from the food pyramid most of us remember learning as a child, but incorporating different food categories (fruits, vegetables, grains, protein, and dairy) remains the science-based recommendation.

Some people have dietary restrictions based on medical issues, religious beliefs, environmental concerns, or considerations of animal treatment. If you follow any modified diet, make sure you do it in a healthy way. I could be vegan by eating only potato chips covered in chocolate syrup all day, every day, but that would be suboptimal for many reasons. Be mindful of what you are putting into your body, and consult with a medical professional for guidance.

> I could be vegan by eating only potato chips covered in chocolate syrup all day, every day, but that would be suboptimal for many reasons.

Protein is important for tissue healing and energy. Most people associate protein with animal products such as meat, eggs, and cheese. For those adhering to meat-free or dairy-free diets, protein can be obtained through tofu, beans, nuts, seeds, and some grains.

Gut inflammation can obstruct healing and contribute to negative mental health effects. Avoid foods that contribute to inflammation, such as white breads and pastas, fried foods, sugar-sweetened beverages, processed meats (such as hot dogs), and processed snack foods. Incorporate anti-inflammatory foods such as whole grains, beans, seeds, nuts, fruits, vegetables, and fish into your diet.

Make sure you are consuming lots of calcium, which is especially important if you are breast- or chestfeeding. Calcium supports bone health for both the baby and you, as your body's estrogen level (which supports bone health) is low during breast- or chestfeeding. If you follow a dairy-free diet or are lactose intolerant, many dairy alternatives (think almond-, coconut-, pea-, or oat-based milks and yogurts) have equal or increased calcium when compared to their dairy-based counterparts.

It's common to become at least slightly anemic in pregnancy, plus everyone loses some blood with delivery. Eating high-iron foods such as meats, tofu, beans, seeds, and spinach can improve your recovery and energy level. You can take an iron supplement (which might be directly recommended by your health care clinician), but be aware that this often contributes to constipation (which we've already covered). If you find yourself constantly desiring to chew on ice, this can be a sign of significant anemia, and you may need more than just iron-rich foods and oral supplements, such as IV iron or a blood transfusion.

Continue consuming fish with caution if you're breast- or chestfeeding, as mercury in fish can pass through the milk and impact the baby's development. The amount of exposure is less than what occurs through the placenta during pregnancy, but you should still try to avoid eating large fish. Small fish such as salmon do not contain high amounts of mercury and can benefit the baby's brain development. If you're not breast- or chestfeeding, go to town on the seafood.

Hot dogs, deli meats, and soft cheese are okay to eat, even if breast- or chestfeeding. The risk of exposing the baby through the milk to the dangerous bacteria *Listeria*, which these foods may contain, is extremely low.

> Eat your fruits and veggies!

If you had gestational diabetes, you are at an increased risk for chronic diabetes. Continue being judicious in your carb intake. You should undergo diabetes testing about six to twelve weeks postpartum, and you should be screened for diabetes every few years after that.

Blood pressure issues in pregnancy increase your risk for lifelong heart disease. Limit excess sugar, salt, and bad fats (saturated and trans fats). Eat your fruits and veggies!

Drink water. This is such a simple part of general health that many people ignore. Juice, soda, and energy drinks can't top that high-quality H_2O.

Caffeine does pass into human-produced milk and, in excessive amounts, can cause a baby consuming that milk to be fussy and irritable and have sleep issues. If breast- or chestfeeding, caffeine should generally be limited to 300 to 750 mg per day. To put that into perspective, an average 8-oz. cup of coffee contains around 100 mg of caffeine, so you still have the opportunity to drink a potentially ridiculous amount of coffee. Please consider all other caffeine sources, including tea, soda, energy drinks, and chocolate. If you avoided caffeine completely during pregnancy, your baby might be more sensitive to it in your milk. If you're not breast- or chestfeeding, just don't drink so much caffeine that you're unable to sleep when needed or that it's causing you any physical symptoms.

> You still have the opportunity to drink a potentially ridiculous amount of coffee.

Vitamins support your health during the postpartum period and can provide a breast- or chestfeeding baby with beneficial nutrients. Either continue your prenatal vitamin or switch to a postnatal vitamin that has additional components.

Now for the million-dollar question: Should you eat your placenta? In the United States, the practice of placental consumption (called placentophagy) was first documented in the 1970s, but it has been a hot topic in recent years. The act is based on the notion that almost all other mammals participate in placentophagy — but keep in mind that animals do an awful lot of things that we don't, and I do mean *awful*.

Advocates of placentophagy also propose its benefits for postpartum energy, mood, pain control, and lactation. There are not great studies in humans nor animals to support these beliefs. When talking about any intervention, we think about both benefits and harms. Placental tissue could potentially retain bacteria or viruses that can pass to the phoenix and to the baby through human milk. In 2017, the Centers for Disease Control and Prevention released a warning about placentophagy after a breastfeeding infant developed sepsis potentially stemming from the practice, although that link could not be confirmed.

Consider also that there are no standards for the sterilization and preparation of placentas for consumption. If you have your placenta made into pills, the most common method, how do you know you're receiving pills filled with your personal placenta, and what else might they contain? In the end, there may or may not be benefits and risks to consuming your placenta. I tell my patients about the lack of evidence, that I personally wouldn't do it, and that the Amer-

ican College of Obstetricians and Gynecologists rec-
ommends against it, and leave them to their own
decisions. If you decide to eat your placenta, have
it prepared by a trusted source and understand the
process of preparation.

In the end, there may or may not be benefits and risks to consuming your placenta.

Some phoenixes appreciate
being able to have an alcoholic
drink again after delivery. Please
be cognizant that regardless of
your previous level of alcohol
consumption, your tolerance is
likely now reduced. Don't over-
do it, both for your health and safety and that of the
baby. You don't want your judgment to be impaired
when you're responsible for a tiny human. If breast-
or chestfeeding, know that alcohol can pass into the
milk and affect the baby. Wait, optimally, three to
four hours — no less than two — per drink to breast-
or chestfeed after alcohol consumption. Pump and
dump if you need to empty your milk prior to that
for comfort. Excessive alcohol use can impact milk
supply and impact the baby's development and sleep
patterns.

It would be silly of me not to talk about marijuana.
Though it's not legal everywhere, there are people
who use it everywhere, including phoenixes. Because use statistics are based on self-reporting, it's

difficult to capture the true incidence, but let's just say it's common. Tetrahydrocannabinol (THC), marijuana's psychoactive component, does pass to infants via human milk. It may impact development, particularly of the brain. Data suggest the possibility of increased anxiety and decreased nutrition in infants exposed to THC through human-produced milk. Marijuana, too, can cloud judgment, and intoxication can ultimately be dangerous to a phoenix as well as a baby in the care of someone who is high. Even slight alterations in the phoenix's mental state or actions can impact bonding and play, subsequently affecting the child's emotional regulation. First- and secondhand marijuana smoke likely has similar detrimental effects to lung health as seen with smoke from nicotine and tobacco cigarettes. If using marijuana, know its source and be aware of its potential to be laced with other drugs.

Cannabidiol (CBD), touted to potentially provide the same medical benefits as marijuana, such as pain control and management of depression without the psychoactive effects, is becoming more popular in even over-the-counter products. CBD has not yet been widely studied and results are not sufficient to recommend use. Many CBD products contain lead and mercury, which can negatively affect adults and children.

I would be remiss not to touch on other substances as well, especially in light of the growing opioid epidemic in the United States. Drug use for recreation and due to addiction is real. Illicit substances have numerous health risks, including death. Please tell your health care clinician about any drug use so the potential impacts can be discussed. If you are struggling with addiction and do not know where to go for help, contact the Substance Abuse and Mental Health Services Administration (SAMHSA) helpline at 1-800-662-HELP (4357).

WARNINGS

- Feeling a strong desire to chew on ice

- Feeling the need to use alcohol, marijuana, or other substances on a daily basis and/or in large amounts

- Impairment of daily function due to substance use

- Persistent feelings of weakness and fatigue

QUESTIONS

- Are there any dietary recommendations for my particular circumstances?

- Which vitamin do you recommend I take?

SUPPLIES

- Prenatal or postnatal vitamins

> *I was worried to talk to most people about it because I was afraid they would think I was being a bad mom or I wasn't able to handle taking care of my child, which wasn't the issue at all.*

Betsy, North Dakota

16

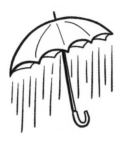

FREE YOUR MIND

Peripartum Mood Disorders

EVEN IN THE best scenarios, phoenixes may experience a broad range of negative mental health effects, including depression, anxiety, and — less commonly — psychosis. Complications or atypical circumstances arising throughout the pregnancy, during the delivery, or postpartum, or if the phoenix has a history of mental health issues, all increase the risk of a peripartum mood disorder.

It is difficult to assess the incidence of these issues, as they are often underreported. This is unsurprising given the strong societal stigma surrounding mental health in general, even more so during and after pregnancy. Based on limited data, about one in seven women will experience postpartum depression.

One phoenix recounted to me her experience with postpartum depression, which still makes her tearful to talk about years after the fact. She remembered crying at seemingly random times throughout the day. It occurred during any activity and was generally unprovoked. When she returned to work, it impacted her ability to complete normal tasks. She also found herself simply not enjoying her work, though she had previously thought of it as her dream job, so she thought about quitting. She recalled sensing that her absence would improve the lives of her friends, family, baby, and coworkers, even though she knew logically this was not true. By allowing and accepting support from her friends and family, participating in counseling, and using an antidepressant medication for a few months, she finally noticed an improvement in her mental health.

> Peripartum mood disorders are NOT a sign that you do not love your baby or that you are a bad person.

Let me be clear: Peripartum mood disorders are NOT a sign that you do not love your baby or that you are a bad person. They are a result of chemical and hormonal factors beyond your control.

SYMPTOMS OF A PERIPARTUM MOOD DISORDER

- Constant worry
- Extreme irritability
- Fear of failing as a parent
- Feelings of hopelessness or worthlessness
- Inability to concentrate
- Insomnia
- Loss of appetite
- Loss of interest and pleasure in previously enjoyable activities
- Overeating
- Racing or obsessive thoughts
- Rapid mood swings
- Sleeping too much
- Thoughts of harm to yourself, your baby, or others
- Uncontrollable crying

The severity, number, and impact of these symptoms are important to consider when sorting out the presence of a peripartum mood disorder. A majority of phoenixes will experience the "baby blues," which involve mild emotional lability, stress, and tearfulness that may last a few days or weeks due to normal changes such as hormone fluctuations, poor sleep, and increased stress. You might need some extra support and can consider counseling for the baby blues, but medication is generally not appropriate or necessary in this setting.

A majority of phoenixes will experience the "baby blues."

If you're worried about any of the symptoms above, don't ignore them. Acknowledging their presence is the first step in managing them.

If you can, optimize your lifestyle as much as possible with healthy eating, exercise, adequate sleep, and help from your support systems. Sometimes these efforts are not sufficient or possible, however.

Talk to your trusted health care professional if you're worried. This might be your prenatal care clinician, your delivery clinician, your primary care clinician (these are not all always the same person!), or some other specialist. It can be easiest to talk about this with someone who knows you well and with whom you feel comfortable being open and honest.

They may refer you to a therapist, counselor, or psychiatrist specializing in peripartum mood disorders. It can do wonders to have an unbiased resource to whom you can vent, cry, scream, and talk things out in whatever way works best for you. Some people do require medications in the short or long term to fully manage their symptoms.

Diagnosing and managing peripartum mood disorders is important to keep you at your healthiest. Don't be afraid to address your mental health concerns.

WARNINGS

- Any of the symptoms listed on page 145

QUESTIONS

- Is what I'm feeling normal, or should I seek help?

- What resources are available for counseling/therapy/support?

- Would you recommend medications for my mental health?

> *I wish I had known about PTSD after NICU. No one ever told me this was something to look out for. I thought I was completely losing my mind when we got home. It was horrible.*

Kelly, Delaware

17

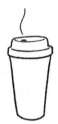

I C U, BB

NICU

I**T IS SO** challenging to have your baby admitted to the neonatal intensive care unit (NICU). Some parents are expecting it due to planned preterm delivery or the baby's known medical problems. Other times, issues arise during labor or delivery or in the neonatal period that weren't predicted. It's okay to struggle with this.

Once your baby is admitted to the NICU, try to mentally prepare yourself prior to heading in for a visit. It can be traumatic to see your baby with an IV, breathing tube, catheter, or monitoring wires.

It can be traumatic to see your baby with an IV, breathing tube, catheter, or monitoring wires.

There will likely be other babies around with similar attachments. Try not to let this scare you. You might not be able to handle it for long right away, and that's okay. It takes time to adjust to this new territory.

Familiarize yourself with the hospital's visitation rules of who can see the baby in the NICU and when. Parents often have 24/7 access, but this isn't always true.

Anyone who visits should wash their hands thoroughly prior to entering the NICU. Hand sanitizer is usually readily available throughout the NICU as well.

Introduce yourself to the medical team and staff. Be present at least occasionally during morning rounds to receive the most thorough updates on your baby's medical requirements and prognosis. Ask questions at this and any time so you can most fully understand the clinical picture.

See if there are portions of care in which you can participate. When babies are very sick, unfortunately phoenixes aren't able to help a lot. Helping with a bath or feeding, however, can be huge. When safely allowable, cradle your baby with skin-to-skin contact. Talk, sing, and read to your baby. Starting a positive relationship with your baby can still happen even if the circumstances aren't as expected.

Make sure to take care of yourself! You will be mainly focused on your baby, but in order to stay healthy for that baby, you must address your own needs — you can't care for others if you don't care for yourself. Drink lots of water, eat when you're hungry, shower, and for goodness's sake, get some sleep. Some hospitals provide special accommodations for NICU parents, but do not underestimate the power of going home to sleep in your own bed.

> Be present at least occasionally during morning rounds to receive the most thorough updates on your baby's medical requirements and prognosis.

Ask NICU and OB staff at your hospital if they can refer you to any local NICU parent support groups. It can be helpful to talk to people who are going through or have gone through a similar situation.

Designate one point person (family or friend) who can disseminate information to others so you aren't pressured to constantly text, call, and email updates to everyone you know. Alternatively or in addition to this, many websites let loved ones access what is essentially your personal blog of the baby's progress.

There are likely to be setbacks and times of status quo with a prolonged NICU stay. Take it day by day, focus on the positives, and celebrate every milestone.

Take pictures! You might not get to have a fancy photo session right away with baby curled up on a blanket in a cute basket, but you will still likely want to hold on to these early memories, no matter what the outcome may be in the end.

Take it day by day and celebrate every milestone.

Having an infant admitted to the NICU can lead to prolonged mental health effects for phoenixes. Some experience constant anxiety about what might happen to their babies in the future. Some feel depressed. Some have post-traumatic stress disorder, recalling what their babies experienced. My friends have told me about being triggered by even subtle scents that remind of them of the NICU stay. Be aware of this possible effect and reach out for help if needed.

The NICU is a hard place to be. Make the best you can of every day.

QUESTIONS

- Are there resources in the community that can help us?

- Can you explain the purpose of each intervention that's happening?

- How can I participate in the baby's care?

- How long do you think each intervention will be needed?

- How might the baby's issues affect him/her long-term?

- Is there a family room at the hospital where we can stay?

- Who can I talk to about finances/insurance for a NICU stay?

- Who can visit the NICU, and when?

Of course I love my baby. We just didn't click right away. It was upsetting not to feel that bond, but it came with time.

Anonymous

18

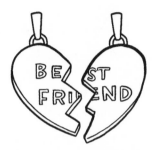

I CAN TELL THAT WE ARE GOING TO BE FRIENDS

Bonding with Baby

YOU MIGHT NOT feel bonded with your baby right away. This is okay. Bonding with your offspring is not necessarily immediate or natural. Feeling like a parent whose whole life has magically changed doesn't happen all at once. Not everyone takes on a nurturing caretaker role effortlessly.

One phoenix told me she hadn't ever considered the possibility of *not* bonding immediately and was surprised, frustrated, and disappointed when it happened between her and her baby. She felt love in an almost mandatory sense but felt hopeless in their lack of connection, as if her baby wasn't even hers. It took months not to feel like she was simply babysitting for a relative and to feel a positive parent-child connection.

> Feeling like a parent whose whole life has magically changed doesn't happen all at once.

Bonding with the baby may take days, weeks, or months. Complications with pregnancy, delivery, or the postpartum period may prolong the process. Sometimes it takes a while even with circumstances that are otherwise seemingly normal. Struggling through this does not make you a bad person or parent — most relationships require some work to get started!

Spending more skin-to-skin contact time with your baby can help with bonding. Cuddling and snuggling won't suddenly transform you, but it can help. Take part in general care, such as feeding, clothing, and changing diapers, rather than deferring these tasks to others. This is a little bit of "fake it 'til you make it," but you don't have to frame it that way. Any goal takes effort. For the most part, though, developing a bond or connection is simply a matter of time.

Try not to compare your relationship with your

baby to the experience of other phoenixes who say they fell in love right away with their babies. Everyone's experience is different. Your baby is absolutely not going to remember this period of time.

> Cuddling and snuggling won't suddenly transform you, but it can help.

QUESTIONS

- Are there community resources that can help me?

- I'm not feeling bonded with the baby. Is this normal at this point? How can I improve this?

It's just such a major transition to go from working fifty-plus hours a week, going to work, then the gym, and maybe meeting friends out to pretty much staying at home and maybe leaving the house once a day. Yes, the baby is amazing and the cuddles are top-notch! But the conversation and intellectual stimulation are not quite the same.

Sam, North Carolina

19

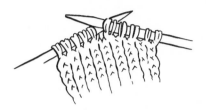

I AM SO LONELY

Social Life

YOUR EXISTING RELATIONSHIPS may be affected by your phoenix status, and your ability to spend time with friends in the same ways you previously did might change. If you have a baby at home, that new person reliant on you will keep you relatively housebound initially. Even though you are physically with a person at almost all times, they're a baby who can't talk back. That doesn't make for the most intellectually stimulating companion. For those who are without a baby for whatever reason, friends and family might not be sure of the best way to support you, which can lead to situations where it seems like they are ignoring or avoiding you. The postpartum period can be isolating, and the loneliness is jarring and intolerable for some phoenixes.

Having a partner or other support person at home with you 24/7 for the first few days or weeks can be helpful on a number of levels. Some phoenixes have the good fortune to have multiple people who are able to do this, and they're able to set up a schedule that extends over weeks to months of who will be around when.

> The postpartum period can be isolating.

Not everyone is so lucky. Call your loved ones for a chat; it's helpful to speak with an adult during or after being alone with an infant and/or your thoughts and emotions all day. Invite friends over to visit when you're ready, but do not feel the need to tidy up or prepare your place for their presence. Take people up on their offers for help and support, such as with grocery shopping or laundry; this is the ultimate version of friends with benefits. Try to get out of the house to meet up for a decently timed meal. Don't feel the need to stay out late into the night, but tailor fun to your new schedule. Go for a walk in your neighborhood with baby in a stroller and simply say hello to passersby. Join in-person or online groups for new parents.

This can also be an excellent time to focus on your

interests and redevelop your relationship with yourself. Read a book you've been meaning to get around to. Get back into an old hobby, such as crocheting. Cook some new recipes for the week's meal prep. Listen to your favorite music and sing your heart out throughout the rest of the day. If you're your only friend for the day, you might as well make yourself good company.

> This can also be an excellent time to focus on your interests and redevelop your relationship with yourself.

Above all, keep in mind that just because your social life may be transiently or permanently different doesn't mean it's over. The friends who are worth it will still be there. You may make new friends. Any friends who abandon you with this new journey may not have been the best friends for you anyway. Thank you, next.

QUESTIONS

- Are there community resources that could help me?

- How can I become involved in new parent groups?

> *The exhaustion doesn't last forever. You will make it through this. I needed to hear that a few times when I had my third week of fifteen-minute cat naps and was too tired to chew.*

Kim, Pennsylvania

20

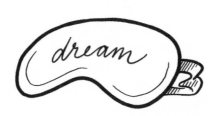

DREAM A LITTLE DREAM

Sleep

AS IF ALL of this isn't difficult enough, you're likely going to be running on a suboptimal amount of sleep in the postpartum period. Phoenixes tend to laugh off questions about sleep, but it's usually obvious that the laughs are a cover for wanting to cry. Essentially, everything we've gone over so far cuts down on your quantity and quality of sleep, and it's all worsened by the fickle needs of babies or by pervasive thoughts about not having a baby at home with you at this time. Sleep deprivation makes normal functioning difficult, harms your long-term health, and contributes to peripartum mood disorders.

Prioritize sleep. Laundry, dishes, elaborate cooking, cleaning, running errands — these things can wait (or be delegated to support people). If you're exhausted and the choice lies between getting some shut-eye and folding towels, please choose the Zs. The towels will be there later (and unfolded towels still work great — just sayin').

> Please choose the Zs.

Don't overextend yourself. Many phoenixes feel the need to return to work too soon, continue with volunteer and side projects while on parental leave, allow too many visitors, or sign up for new parent/baby classes and groups. These things can be good in moderation, but there's no reason to fill every minute of your daily schedule. Don't make yourself participate in so many typically fun, positive, and otherwise helpful activities that it exhausts you and cuts down on the number of hours left to even try to sleep.

If you have duties you absolutely must attend to, do what you can to multitask when you're awake so your mental to-do list isn't distracting you from the sleep you need later. Dance for exercise with the baby in a carrier while you talk on the phone with a friend while washing dishes while a load of laundry is in the dryer. Okay, maybe it's ambitious to think the stars can align for that scenario to be a reality, but you get the idea.

Create a plan with any available support people about sharing responsibilities both day and night. Take people up on their offers for help. Maybe your partner or support person can take charge of a night-time feeding so you can get a longer stretch of sleep. Maybe a relative can watch the baby during the day while you shower and take some time alone so you don't have to do those things later while the baby is sleeping.

One phoenix told me through tears that she was averaging three hours of sleep, separated into short spurts, in each twenty-four-hour period. The

> Take people up on their offers for help.

baby was colicky and having difficulty feeding. The phoenix's partner was having a hard time coming to terms with parenthood and was not participating in almost any baby care or household chores. After they had an honest conversation and additionally received some help from family, the phoenix's sleep improved considerably.

If you can, sleep when the baby sleeps. This can be impossible for some, and those phoenixes would laugh in my face. At least try.

Avoid activities in your bed other than sleep. When your mind is trained that your bed is for sleeping, it can be easier to fall asleep when needed. If you read, eat, scroll on your phone, watch TV, or anything else in bed, it becomes an alert activity zone instead.

Above all, keep in mind: it gets better.

Sometimes, phoenixes do need medications to help with sleep. Be very cautious with sleep medications in general, given potential side effects or dependency. This is especially important if you have any responsibility for a baby after taking the medication. Over-the-counter sleep aids such as Unisom can knock you out for seven to eight hours (or more). Although that amount of sleep may sound nice, it may be counterproductive to other goals, such as breast- or chestfeeding or pumping during the night. Some prescription sleep medications have contributed to sleepwalking and bizarre (even dangerous) sleep behavior. Talk to your health care clinician if you feel you may need sleep medications.

WARNINGS

- Complete lack of sleep

- Not feeling rested after at least seven hours of sleep

- Sleeping most hours of the day

QUESTIONS

- How can I improve my sleep?

- Is the amount of sleep I'm getting normal and okay?

SUPPLIES

- Aromatherapy

- Blackout curtains

- Sleep sound machine

> *Don't try to do it all
> when you get home! Get help.
> Your main job is to feed the baby
> and take care of yourself. Let
> everyone else help with the other
> stuff, if possible. The first month
> feels like a daze.*

Patricia, Nevada

21

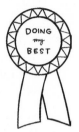

WE'RE GOING TO MAKE IT AFTER ALL

Other Tips

WE'VE GONE THROUGH tearing, incisions, bleeding, cramping, peeing, pooping, hemorrhoids, exercise, body changes, sex, birth control, feeding, eating, mood disorders, NICU struggles, infant bonding, social life changes, sleeping, and more. What a party!

SOME OTHER TIPS AND THOUGHTS

- Unfollow or mute any social media account that brings negative energy into your life. Social media often inaccurately represents reality, instead portraying a filtered idealization. Catching a glimpse of some perfectly styled and posed postpartum family that seemingly has everything together? You don't need that.

- On a similar note, don't compare yourself to other phoenixes (friends, coworkers, family members, neighbors, celebrities). Everyone has a different journey.

- Keep a journal/diary/blog of what you're going through. It can be therapeutic for you and helpful to you or others in the future.

- If you're interested and able, hire out help. Get a neighbor kid to mow the lawn. Pay the extra price for grocery delivery. Have a cleaning service come by even just once. It will feel like a mini vacation to relieve yourself of those responsibilities.

- See what professional medical help is available to you at home. Some obstetric clinicians are able to do home visits after delivery. In many areas, phoenixes can schedule visiting nurses to stop in for health assessments. Lactation consultants and postpartum doulas can assist with breast- or chestfeeding support and general care.

- Get some fresh air at least once a day. That can be as simple as sitting outside for a feeding sesh. (If it's the dead of winter in a frigid area, maybe just hang out by a window.)

- Positive affirmations can be helpful. Once a day or week, acknowledge your successes, no matter how seemingly small or insignificant.

- If you had a job prior to delivery and are planning to ultimately return to work, maximize your leave. You'll never get that time back. Make sure you are extremely comfortable with the childcare you've arranged thereafter.

- Give yourself permission to not be okay.

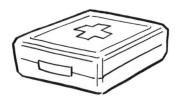

22

POSTPARTUM SURVIVAL KIT

Supplies

HERE'S A LIST of all of the supplies suggested throughout the guide. Have these items ready for when you get home after delivery.

- Abdominal binder
- Access to a media streaming service
- Acetaminophen
- Adult diapers
- Aromatherapy
- Blackout curtains
- Bottle brush

- Bottle drying rack
- Bottles and nipples
- Breast or chest pump
- Comfortable and supportive sports bra
- Comfortable exercise clothing
- Epsom salt
- Fenugreek supplements
- Fiber-rich snacks
- Formula
- Formula coupons
- Good book
- Gym membership or home exercise equipment (even if that's just walking shoes!)
- Heating pad or a sock full of rice to warm in the microwave
- Hemorrhoid cream
- Ibuprofen
- Ice packs
- Incontinence pantyliners
- Lotion

- Lounging pants

- Lube

- Nipple cream

- Nipple shields

- Nonfluoridated water

- Overnight menstrual pads

- Pantyliners

- Phone apps

- Pillow

- Prenatal or postnatal vitamins

- Regular menstrual pads

- Sleep sound machine

- Spray bottle

- Stool softener

- Sunflower lecithin

- Throwaway underwear

- Tucks pads

- Vitamins

- Water

- Witch hazel

I tried to schedule an appointment four weeks postpartum because I had some questions and because that was when I had childcare, as my mom was in town. I was told it was emergency department (ED) or wait until six weeks. I waited until six, as ED seemed like overkill, but then had to bring my newborn with me. I spent less than ten minutes with my OB and basically didn't ask questions because my kiddo was crying, so I couldn't focus enough on me to even read the prepared list of questions I had.

Nichole, Michigan

23

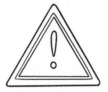

KEEP AWAY FROM THE DANGER

Emergencies

'VE MENTIONED SYMPTOMS to watch for and topics to discuss with your health care professional throughout this guide. Not all these are emergent issues that need attention right away. I've listed the most pressing symptoms below. Please contact a health care professional if you experience any of the following issues. They may be symptoms of an underlying problem that needs to be addressed, and the symptoms themselves may compromise your health. You may need to advocate hard for yourself to get an appointment, depending on how your preferred health care clinician's office operates. Know that an urgent care facility or emergency room is always an option if you are concerned and unable to get an appointment. Yes, costs go up in that situation, but your health and safety are a priority.

WARNINGS

- Any pain not controlled with oral medications

- Bleeding through more than one pad in an hour persistently

- Chest pain

- Discharge or bleeding from a C-section incision

- Inability to have a bowel movement or pass gas

- Inability to urinate

- Passing clots larger than the size of lemons

- Persistent headache

- Persistent pain in the upper abdomen

- Separation of the C-section incision

- Shortness of breath

- Significant swelling of an extremity

- Spots, flashes, or blind areas in visual fields

- Temperature > 100.4 degrees Fahrenheit

- Thoughts of harm to yourself, your baby, or others

- Uncontrollable vomiting/inability to keep down food or fluids

- Urethral pain with urination

- Vaginal discharge with a bad odor or abnormal color

QUESTIONS

- When should I follow up postpartum?

- If I have a problem sooner than that, who should I call/where should I go?

The intersection between mama's issues and baby's issues when it comes to breastfeeding can be confusing. I know there are a lot of resources out there for these things, but that can be overwhelming too. Even just a list of all the things the OB/GYN can address during the postpartum period would be helpful because it's broader than just issues related to the physical recovery from giving birth.

Kristin, Minnesota

24

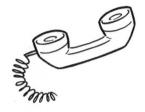

WHO YOU GONNA CALL?

Contacts

IT CAN BE difficult to know where to turn when post-partum concerns arise, and you want to go to the correct source for answers. For example, although OB/GYNs receive a broad general medical education prior to our specialized training, our main skill set when it comes to babies is safely assisting their exit from the uterus and promptly handing them off to someone else. We don't have the best answers for caring for the baby after that.

Call your obstetrics clinician (the person who cared for you in pregnancy) with:

- Concerns about your own physical or mental health

- Need for advice for any activity/exposure restrictions or recommendations for you

- Questions about breast- or chestfeeding (particularly regarding ways to increase supply or concerns for possible development of clogged ducts or mastitis)

- Questions about medications you can take

- Requests for referral physical therapy or other care

Call your pediatrician (the person who cares for your baby) with:

- Concerns about the baby's health

- Need for advice for any activity/exposure restrictions or recommendations for the baby

- Questions about breast- or chestfeeding (particularly regarding baby's latch or assessment of baby's intake)

- Questions about formula-feeding

- Questions about medications the baby can receive

Call your non-obstetrics primary care clinician (the person who cares for your general medical issues) with:

- Concerns about your own physical health that you are 100-percent sure are unrelated to the fact that a baby recently came out of you (earache, for example)*

Call your lactation consultant (the person who gives you advice on breast- or chestfeeding, if you have one) with:

- Questions about breast- or chestfeeding (particularly tips and tricks on the process itself, but really any question could be fair game here)

- Questions about medications you can take while breast- or chestfeeding

---

*You can call your obstetrics clinician about these types of problems too, but you're probably going to get the most appropriate evaluation and management plan from your primary care clinician, and some patients logistically have an easier time making an appointment/being assessed promptly for these types of issues in a non-obstetrics office.

25

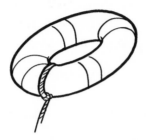

HELP ME IF YOU CAN

Resources

T HESE ARE SOME great online resources that may help you in your recovery.

• **The 4th Trimester Project (www.jordanin-stituteforfamilies.org/innovate/4thtrimester-project)** aims to improve the time after delivery.

• **The American College of Obstetricians and Gynecologists (www.acog.org)** is the largest organization of OB/GYNs in the United States that provides OB/GYNs guidelines for all areas of OB/GYN practice. ACOG also supplies patient education materials on many topics.

- **BabyCenter (www.babycenter.com/postpartum-health)** is an online community for pregnancy, postpartum, and parenting support.

- **Bedsider (www.bedsider.org/methods)** is a fantastic resource for comparing contraceptive methods to figure out which might be best for you.

- **The Academy of Breastfeeding Medicine (www.bfmed.org)** is an international organization of physicians focused on supporting and promoting breast- or chestfeeding.

- **BirthFit (www.birthfit.com)** focuses on nutrition and exercise for conception, pregnancy, and postpartum.

- **The Blue Dot Project (www.thebluedot-project.org)** was created to raise awareness of, reduce stigma surrounding, and provide support for postpartum mental health issues.

- **The Centers for Disease Control and Prevention (www.cdc.com)** is a national public health institute. Its website provides information on breast- or chestfeeding, formula-feeding, nutrition, postpartum mental health, and much more.

- **DONA International (www.dona.org/what-is-a-doula/find-a-doula)**, formerly Doulas of North America, can help you find a postpartum doula in your area.

- **Faces of Loss, Faces of Hope (www.facesofloss.com)** provides support and resources to those experiencing pregnancy or infant loss.

- **FC2 (www.fc2.us.com)** is the internal condom.

- **Kelly Mom (www.kellymom.com)** was started by a lactation consultant to provide evidence-based information on many breast- or chestfeeding-related topics.

- **KidsHealth (www.kidshealth.org/en/parents/pregnancy-newborn/formulafeed)** provides information on formula-feeding at every stage.

- **La Leche League International (www.llli.org)** is a nonprofit focused on advocacy, education, and training to support breast- or chestfeeding.

- **Moms on Call (www.momsoncall.com)** has videos and merchandise that help with infant care.

- **MUTU System (www.mutusystem.com)** is an exercise program to improve pelvic floor and abdominal strength and healing.

- **The National Domestic Violence Hotline (www.thehotline.org/1-800-799-7233)** is available 24/7 and offers tools and help to victims to build lives free of domestic abuse.

- **Postpartum Support International (www. postpartum.net)** provides mental health resources for postpartum individuals.

- **The Postpartum Health Alliance (www.postpartumhealthalliance.org)** aims to increase awareness and support for peripartum mood disorders.

- **Postpartum Progress (www.postpartumprogress.com)** is a widely read blog about postpartum mental health.

- **Reddit (www.redditcom/r/mommit, www. reddit.com/r/beyondthebump)** is an online aggregate of news, social media, opinion, and much more. It is a collection of subreddits, forums for specific content areas. r/Mommit and r/beyondthebump are focused on pregnancy, postpartum, and parenting.

- **Romper (www.romper.com)** bills itself as the "leading digital destination for millennial moms."

- **ScaryMommy (www.scarymommy.com)** is an online community primarily directed at parenthood but contains content on much more.

- **The Substance Abuse and Mental Health Services Administration (www.samhsa. gov/find-help/national-helpline)** can help connect anyone to local substance abuse and mental health resources.

- **"This is Postpartum" by Meg Boggs Blog (www.facebook.com/megboggsblog/videos/230445860960929)** is an empowering video that shows many phoenixes talking about their postpartum bodies.

It is worthwhile to let those you love see you struggle and not try to hide it. I try to make it reaffirming that you will, inevitably, lose your shit. It happens to us all. Hormones are legit.

THE best sage advice I ever got: "The baby has no idea that you don't know what you are doing."

Jodi, Vermont

AFTERBIRTH

AS I SAID in the beginning, this guide is by no means all-encompassing. One book can't change the world, and I have no grand expectations of fixing the entirety of the "postpartum problem" with what I've written here. I hope, though, that this guide can serve as a quick and easy reference to help navigate some of the most common, troubling postpartum issues and help you live your best possible postpartum life. I hope it encourages you to be open and honest about your experience not only with health care professionals but with your friends, family, other people who are important to you, and even strangers. I hope it helps you feel less alone and unsure throughout this time.

The postpartum experience is unique to each individual, but no matter what your particular struggles may be, you are a glorious phoenix. RISE.